Fitness Independence

By Matt Schifferle

Text Copyright © 2016 Matthew J. Schifferle
All Rights Reserved

Ebook ISBN: 9780692744567

Paperback ISBN: ISBN-13:978-1535004220

ISBN-10:1535004223

The information provided in this book is designed to provide helpful information on the subjects discussed. This book is not meant to be used, nor should it be used, to diagnose or treat any medical condition. For diagnosis or treatment of any medical problem, consult your own physician. The publisher and author are not responsible for any specific health or allergy needs that may require medical supervision and are not liable for any damages or negative consequences from any treatment, action, application or preparation, to any person reading or following the information in this book. References are provided for informational purposes only and do not constitute endorsement of any websites or other sources. Readers should be aware that the websites listed in this book may change.

To my Mom, Dad, my Sister Jody and my closest friends, Nicki and Chris.
Thank you for supporting/ putting up with me all as I struggled to figure this stuff out.

Table of Contents

Introduction 5

Part I: Deconstructing The Fitness Lifestyle 7

    1: The True Cost of Fitness 8

    2: The Source of Fitness Success 14

    3: Surface Influences 21

Part II: Basic Principles 29

    4: The Cause of Body Fat 30

    5: The Cause of Training Muscle 48

    6: The Cause of Bodybuilding / Shaping 61

    7: The Cause of Healthy Eating 83

    8: The Delta Principles 99

Part III: Taking Action 118

    9: The Principle Governing Personal Change 119

    10: Building a Plan That Works for You 132

    11: Delta Fitness Methods 151

Introduction

This book is not just about fitness. It's not just a book about six pack abs, building strong muscles or decreasing your body fat percentage. This book is about something much more than getting in shape. This book is about Fitness Independence.

Freedom is the ultimate human pursuit. It's the rallying cry behind revolutions and civil wars. It's also the motivation behind dreams of wealth and financial independence. Just imagine what your life would be like if you never had to worry about money. What sort of work would you do? How would you spend your time? What burdens would you remove? It's not enough to have a lot of money. Without personal freedom, all of the wealth of the world still falls short in bringing personal happiness and fulfillment.

There is a lot of information available about how to become financially independent; to have both money *and* freedom. Unfortunately, there is almost no information on how to be fit and healthy while allowing personal freedom and lifestyle flexibility. While most people admit that compromising one's quality of life for wealth may not be ideal, this notion is not very common when it comes to fitness. In many ways, it's just the opposite. When you read magazines or surf fitness websites, the implied message is that living for the ideal body is the pinnacle of not only a healthy life, but a happy one as well. All around us, the message shouts out "if you dedicate your life towards staying in shape all of your problems will be solved. You'll be healthy, happy and everything will be great." Some experts even claim your diet alone should become an entire lifestyle in its own right! It's a very convincing sales pitch, but it's hiding a dark side. Just as only making a lot of money can't guarantee your happiness, having the body of your dreams at the cost of your quality of life will also be a hollow victory. There are plenty of folks who are in fantastic shape, yet they are still living a very high-stress lifestyle that handicaps their personal happiness. I should know as I used to live that way for many years.

My name is Matt Schifferle, and I once believed that getting in shape was the key to happiness. I fell for the idea that possessing a fit body would give me the life I wanted. Over the years, I realized that the more I pursued this fitness dream, the more my quality of life suffered. My goal of getting in fantastic shape had become my personal nightmare. It took me almost 15 years to learn what was missing. Sure I was lean and muscular, but that wasn't making me happy because it came at the cost of my lifestyle freedom. The more I tightened down my diet and forced myself to hit the gym, the more I felt caged in by my fitness habits. Eventually, I came to crave a different type of fitness lifestyle. I wanted both a fit body and a flexible lifestyle to maintain it. Finally, I learned that fitness is supposed to enhance one's life, not take it over. What use is becoming super fit if you have to dedicate your lifestyle towards struggling to exercise and eat right?

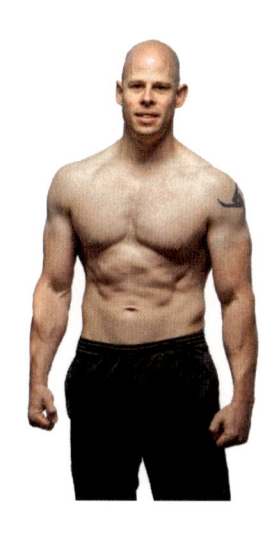

It's this underlying philosophy which motivated me to collect the information in this book. I didn't spend the past ten years writing these pages to help you get in the best shape of your life.

I've written this so you can get in great shape without having to adopt habits that compromise your quality of life.

Just imagine what your life would be like if you never had to worry about missing a workout, or how long you could stay on a diet? How would you live each day if you didn't have to stress over how food is prepared at a restaurant? How much money would you save if you never needed to join a gym? How much time would you save if you no longer had to learn the latest fads and trends?

There are those who will say that such a thing isn't possible, that the straight and narrow is the only way, but this is not at all true. What I've discovered is that not only can you get in shape while maintaining your personal freedom, but you'll probably get even *better* results than ever before.

Personally, I don't practice most of the conventional rules of fitness. I don't do cardio, I don't stretch, and I don't even eat right. I don't need a gym membership nor do I use supplements or spend my time and money reading magazines. To the casual observer, I don't do all that much. The funny thing is I'm in the best shape of my life *because* I break the rules of conventional fitness rather than in spite of it. Results do not have to come at the cost of your lifestyle freedom. Instead, the more liberty and flexibility you enjoy the more potential you will gain!

This book is divided into three sections. The first section pulls back the curtain on the truth about what an exercise lifestyle costs you, and the real factors behind your potential to reach success. The second section is about the rock-bottom rules that govern the results you want. The third section teaches you how to apply those rules in your own way so you can get the best results possible in a way that fits you and your lifestyle like a glove.

It's a great privilege and pleasure to present this information to you. Everything in this book has given me both the fitness I want as well as the lifestyle freedom I need. It's my sincere wish that it can do the same for you.

Part I:
Deconstructing The Fitness Lifestyle

1: The True Cost of Fitness

When I first started working out, I took advantage of low-cost methods like push-ups and jogged around my neighborhood. I even saved money since I wasn't buying junk food after school each day. With these habits, I thought fitness was a free ride.

As it turned out, my lifestyle ended up costing me *a lot*. Within a few months, my diet and exercise plans were consuming my time, effort, discipline, energy, and willpower. By the end of the summer, I was mentally and physically broke. I didn't understand it then, but diet and exercise habits can be incredibly expensive even if they don't hit your wallet. There's a lot more to life

Can you spend your way to a fit body?

Each fitness habit taxes what I call "lifestyle resources." These include any resource you have an infinite supply that influences your quality of life—for example, time, physical energy, emotional energy, willpower, discipline, mental focus, money, and even your living space are all lifestyle resources. A weight machine not only costs you money to acquire it, but it also uses the time it takes to assemble it, maintain it, clean it, and use it. It also costs you the space in your home. So even if you get it on sale, you still pay far more than what's on the price tag.

When running a business or personal budget, it's easy to understand the value of efficient spending. Even the most carefree business owner knows they can't spend too much, or they'll go out of business. However, when it comes to fitness, the common message is "spend, spend, and spend some more!" If you invest more, you'll supposedly gain more, and if that's not the case, it's because you're not spending enough.

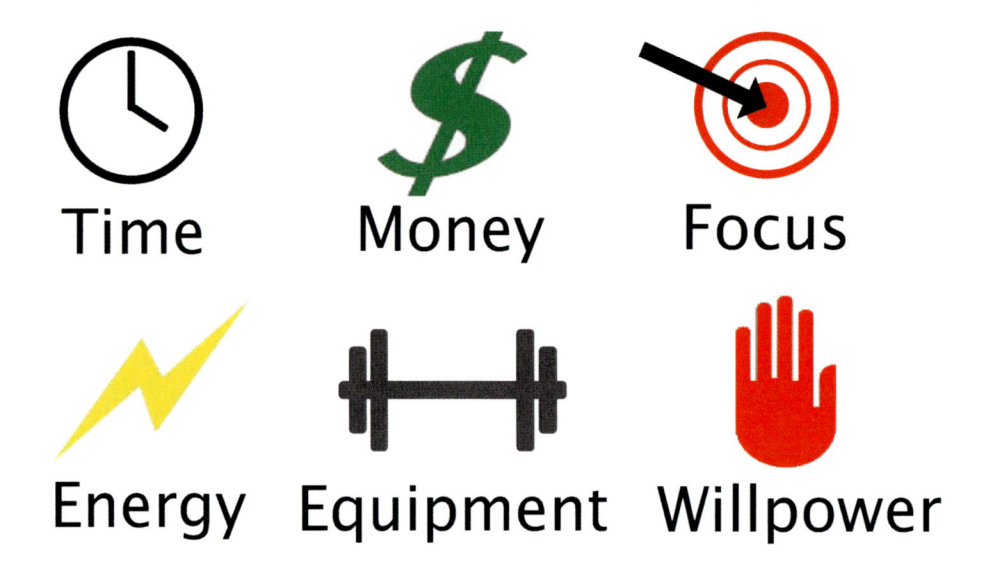

Some of the most common lifestyle resources.

At first, the spend-more-get-more theory works. When you're starting out, an increase in spending will produce results simply because you're going from doing very little to doing a lot more. The downside is this situation has a rapid diminishing rate of return. You don't have unlimited time or energy to hit the gym and ratchet down your diet. Every additional ounce of effort you put into your fitness increases the cost you must pay in lifestyle resources.

The relentless pressure to invest more of yourself is the primary reason why getting in shape can be so incredibly stressful. By far, the biggest source of modern-day stress is stretching the limits of your resources. When you're low on money, you stress over paying the rent on time. Running low on time can make you stress out over being late for an appointment. Running low on emotional energy and willpower means you can't fight off even small temptations, and then you berate yourself for "slipping" off the wagon. Low physical energy means your body can't fight infections, and you often have to resort to habits that tax your joints and organs, causing pain and discomfort. While many claim the rewards of a healthy lifestyle can be yours if you only spend more resources, overspending is a sure way to make you tired and stressed. Overextending yourself is a one-way ticket to poor health rather than a wealth of fitness.

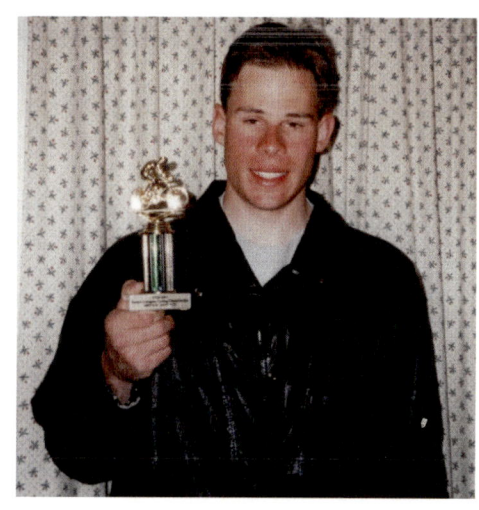

The fatigue on my face shows how tired I was after dedicating my life to bike racing in college. All I did was ride, race and study.

If there's one sure way to ease stress in your life, it's to live below your means. Not just financially but also in your schedule and energy use. If you always leave a little left over you have a buffer that allows you to better handle the challenges of life. Despite the need for efficiency, the message in our fitness culture is that you're not doing enough unless you give everything you've got to your diet and exercise habits. The more you spend and sacrifice the better. It's even admirable to make fitness a source of stress because it means you're doing every little thing you can. People love to brag about how hard they are working and sacrificing in the name of fitness. It's time to change this! Trying to go full tilt all of the time is not the path to success. If you're constantly living on the edge, you won't have any buffer to weather the challenges in life that are sure to crop up. What's even worse is that overextending yourself makes it almost impossible to grow and progress. Once you've used up all of your resources, you cease to move forward just like when you run out of gas in your car.

What's more vexing is everything else in your life also requires your lifestyle resources. Your job, friends, family and other interests also eat up your lifestyle resources. Chances are pretty good these things are also a higher priority than your workout and are costing you most of your resources.

Chances are, you're already maxed out on at least a few of your lifestyle resources. Life has a way of taking up your time and energy just by living it. As great as being lean and healthy is, it's simply not a top priority for most of us above our job, friends, family and everything else.

Despite this, the message still stays the same. Our fitness culture loves to pressure you into spending more lifestyle resources on diet and exercise. You're supposed to make "sacrifices" which is another way of saying "don't spend your lifestyle resources on what you want, spend it on this diet or exercise program instead." It's the fitness equivalent of the corporate rat race.

This free spending is how a few simple, healthy habits can overtake your life. A fitness lifestyle is one where so many resources are spent towards staying in shape that it's the primary focus of your life, and there's not much left for anything else. There's nothing wrong with a diet and exercise lifestyle. If you're an athlete, model or fitness professional then that's great. I don't want to tell anyone how they should live. The only thing is not everyone is going to have the interest, nor the resources, to make fitness the focus of their daily life. Saying most people should adopt a fitness lifestyle to stay in shape is like saying that everyone needs to buy a high-end sports car to get around town. It's fine for some; a few people will bust their tail and make it happen, but most folks will simply not bother and figure they won't ever afford the high cost.

Fitness and Technology

One of the biggest fitness lessons I ever learned was when I visited the Computer History Museum in Silicon Valley. As I walked through the museum, I couldn't help but notice how early computers played a similar role in society that fitness does now. Back then computers were big, complicated and expensive. As a result, Many people wouldn't use a computer unless their job required it. The only other folks who used computers were those who did so because it was a hobby or personal interest. Of course, things changed very quickly as tech giants like Microsoft, Apple and Google hit the computer industry like a tidal wave. Within a few decades, computers were in every home, and everyone was doing their homework on a word processor. Computers went from an obscure part of society to infiltrating every aspect of our lives. As I left the museum and walked past the Google campus, I wondered how such a revolution could take place. The answer was obvious as I thumbed through web pages on my iPhone.

The technological explosion was possible because the lifestyle resources required to buy, use and operate technology have been continuously shrinking. As the lifestyle costs of computers dropped more and more people could use the technology. It spawned innovation and flexibility allowing technology to become the powerful force it is today.

When I came to this realization, I was suddenly aware of how fitness today is just like the early days of computer technology. It's still a high-cost undertaking and as such, most of the folks who pursue fitness do so either because of their profession or because it's a hobby. Sure things like gyms and fat loss programs have grown like crazy

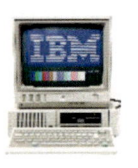

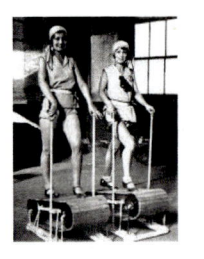

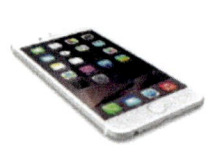

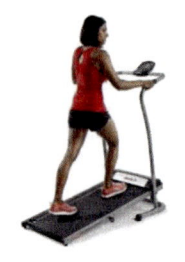

Then   Now

Why has technology become more powerful while staying in shape is still a struggle?

over the past 30 years, but the growth is still within a small segment of society. The reason why staying fit and healthy is such a challenge in our modern society is because we've made fitness an extremely costly undertaking while activities that prevent healthy habits keep getting cheaper. Why should someone spend $100 a month on a gym membership when they can get 300 cable channels for $29? Why spend the time and energy learning how to cook a healthy dinner when you can have take-out delivered to your door in 15 minutes? It's not a question of what's healthier or better for us, but what is easier and less costly to do.

Another parallel is the how computer technology has become more ingrained into everyday life. Computers used to be limited in their application, so they weren't all that important to most people. These days, It doesn't matter what your hobby or profession is, you probably use a computer to some capacity. We've gone from basic tasks like word processing and playing simple games to "there's an app for that" making the computer play a role in everything from building a house to buying coffee.

Sadly, fitness still has a limited application or at least perceived use. Many people don't consider getting in shape important because they "are not that sort of person" and don't care about being able to do things like run long distances or lift heavy weights. So even though a healthy body can improve anyone's quality of life, it's still perceived as a niche interest. These days you don't have to be "into computers" to still use and benefit greatly from them.

Unfortunately, fitness is still publicly perceived as something you need to "be into" to practice it.

Ever since that trip to the Computer History Museum I look at the latest advancements and think to myself "That new computer is amazing......and fitness is still back in the era of the Commodore 64 and Atari." Our current fitness culture is desperately in need of an efficiency upgrade, and this book is where it starts.

Fitness security

The high cost of fitness doesn't just make getting results harder. It also makes it a massive challenge to *maintain* those results as well. Make no mistake about it; you need to pay the cost of staying in shape day after day, month after month and year after year. It's not like buying a material product where you can pay once and then own the thing for life. Once you've paid the price for the fit body, you have to continue paying the cost to maintain the results. So even if the price of a diet or workout is affordable for a short period that still isn't be good enough. The only way you can maintain, a decent level of fitness is if the lifestyle costs of the results are affordable for an extended period. That way, life can't get in the way of you achieving the results you want while also allowing you to keep them as well.

Having a high maintenance fitness lifestyle is usually possible for short periods of time, but the changes in life can make it almost impossible to maintain. If life didn't change, your lifestyle resources would always be consistent. Of course, life does change. One day you can afford a golf club membership and 5 hours on the weekend and the next you're broke and turning your weekends into work-ends. Change is inevitable. If you're going to have any hope of achieving and maintaining your results, you need to make it secure against the natural fluctuations in your lifestyle resources.

Fitness Independence is the art and science of getting the absolute best results through the most efficient use of your lifestyle resources. By keeping the lifestyle costs low, you open up the potential to gain far better results, with much more flexibility, widespread lifestyle application, and the security to know you can maintain your results no matter what life throws at you.

The truth behind excuses

Many fitness experts decry the idea of excuses. They say that we shouldn't make them and that none of the reasons such as a lack of time or energy is a good reason to hide behind. It's as if they expect us just to snap our fingers and somehow wish them away.

The thing is, excuses have a grain of truth to them, and they are most certainly legitimate concerns. These reasons for a lack of progress are not always signs of weakness or a lack of discipline. They are proof that our fitness culture is making diet and exercise far too expensive.

As a trainer, I hear excuses every day as to why people can't do something. Every excuse is a statement about a lack of a resource. People tell me they don't have the time, money, energy or other resources. Making an excuse is just another way of saying that the costs are too high to justify taking action.

The challenge with fitness is you always have to pay the costs up front. You can't get the benefits without spending the resources first. There is no buy-now-pay-later line of fitness credit. What's more vexing is that the benefits are often unique and personal to the individual. As such, the person has little to no way of knowing what the benefits will be. If someone has always suffered from weak legs, then it's going to be a tough sell to convince them to spend the costs to make their legs stronger. They have no idea what developing powerful legs will do for them. It's not like the supermarket where I can give out free samples to entice them to buy the product.

In light of this, it's no wonder why fitness can be such a hard sell. Telling someone to pay the costs for an unknown benefit is quite the uphill battle. Selling healthy habits can be difficult when the prices are high, and the benefits are unknown. Imagine if I came up to you and offered to sell you food you've never eaten for $1,000. I could say anything, but all you'll hear is "Here's a great thing and I promise you'll like it. So how about giving me a lot of money for it right now and it might come to you in 6-8 weeks?"

Plus, that's just for those who are new to fitness. Many folks have a history of trying to get in shape, but their efforts did not produce the results they wanted. Naturally, they stopped paying the cost to maintain the habits that were simply not worth the price. For these people, convincing them they need to spend the necessary costs can be even tougher. They know it wasn't worth it in the past, so why should they try now? Think of a time when someone offered to sell you something, and you said you didn't have the money to afford it. Chances are you could have found a way to afford it. You may have even had the ability to buy it right then, but what you meant was you didn't *want* to spend the money to buy it. There's nothing wrong with that, and that's what is challenging most folks when it comes to getting in shape. They may have the time and energy, but the simple fact is they don't see the value in spending the resources. The costs are too high, and the perceived benefits are too small and uncertain.

The strategies in this book are all designed to help you minimize the risk of investing your resources and maximizing your potential return. It won't cost you much to get started, and the rewards should come rather quickly. They may not start off as massive, changes, but they will at least allow you to dip your toes in the water before deciding you want to go deeper. You don't have to jump in over your head right away and pray you learn how to swim.

A little later on I'll look at more detail at how to tip the tables on this conundrum but for now the take home this simple message: The problem isn't sugar, TV, or desk jobs. We're not fighting an obesity epidemic just because of processed foods or a problem with our healthcare system. All of those things are mere details in light of the simple fact that our fitness culture, and the fitness rat race, has made fitness a high-cost, high-risk, and low-yield endeavor. We are spending lifestyle resources we have in short supply, and the results are often just not worth it.

2: The Source of Fitness Success

I once heard a story of a college professor who put a few large rocks into a glass jar. He held up the jar and asked the students if the jar was full. They all nodded and said yes. He then poured a bag of pebbles into the jar which filled in the cracks between the big rocks. He then did the same thing with sand that filled in the spaces between the stones and finally water which filtered into the sand.

The lesson for the class was that there was always room for more understanding and learning. I took a different lesson away from the story. Those big rocks were the most influential in filling up space in the jar. I saw a direct parallel to this when it came to fitness. At the time, I was juggling many small diet and exercise habits. I figured it would be easier, and more efficient, to just focus on a few big habits as opposed to a bunch of smaller ones. The trick was to figure out what rules and principles were the "big rocks" and the smaller stones that didn't do much.

As I started to question all of my habits I realized most of the newer modern practices didn't have much of an impact. The latest articles in a monthly magazine or blog post were like little grains of sand in that jar. They weren't worthless, but they were too small to produce much of an effect. Meanwhile, the bigger rocks were methods and tactics that had been around for a few generations. If an exercise had lasted 100 years, then it was more basic and fundamental towards primary fitness goals. Most of the trivial trends that existed back in the day had been weeded out through time because they weren't all that important.

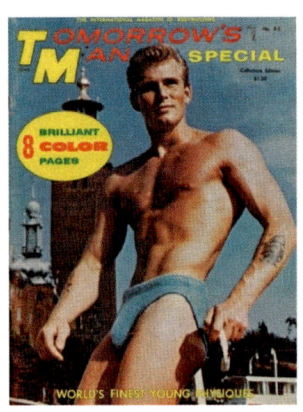

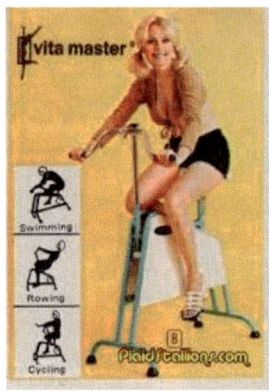

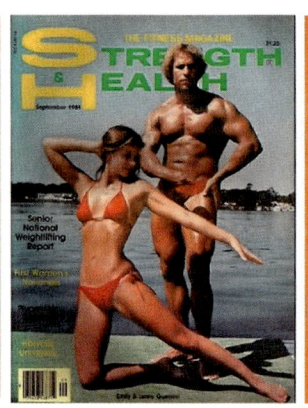

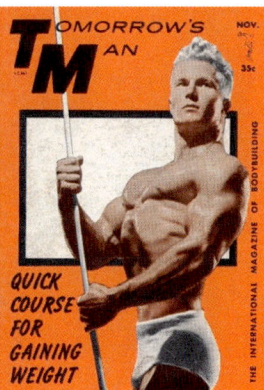

Most diet and exercise methods have only been around for a few decades. These "old school" periodicals are only a single generation old.

Over time, I developed a taste for old school fitness methods. I started learning about the pioneers of our fitness culture who worked out with big heavy barrels and drank whole milk long before weight machines and protein shakes. The classic methods seemed to work, and work very well, yet no one at that time was concerned with the trivial details our modern fitness culture felt was so important. Those old methods were incredibly useful, but more importantly, they were simple and very efficient as well.

Down I dug into the past of our fitness culture. I kept going back further and further like a patient under hypnosis regressing into past lives. Eventually, I started doing research that pre-dated our fitness culture itself. I began looking into the raw science of how and why our body would change even before we knew what a carbohydrate was or before the existence of gyms. I learned that while many think of physical fitness as a natural process, fitness as we practice it is primarily man-made. Furthermore, most of our fitness cultures, even the "old school" stuff has only been in existence for a few decades. Even some of the most traditional methods are just barely 100 years old. The natural laws controlling how your body looks and performs have been in place for eons. However, the rules of diet and exercise people have been using to harness those natural laws are still crude and undeveloped.

I started to ask myself; what is left once you strip everything away? What would be left If you eradicated every modern diet and exercise rule that's popular today? Even without the latest trends, your body would still possess the ability to become lean, strong and fit. So if all of that recent stuff like supplements or cardio machines is not essential, then what is? It was this sort of question that drove me to discover what I like to call the root causes.

> *What we are after is the root and not the branches.*
>
> *The root is the real knowledge; the branches are surface knowledge. Real knowledge breeds "body feel" and personal expression; surface knowledge breeds mechanical conditioning and imposing limitation and squelches creativity.*
> **- Bruce Lee**

What is a cause? Simple, it's the single natural law that is 100% responsible for creating a particular result in your life. It is the rock bottom reason why your body changes and why it's in the current condition it's in right now. It's a natural law untouched by the imagination of man, and thus it doesn't have a bunch of costly rules cluttering it up. Once you understand the cause of your goal you know how to tap into the very heart of what's most important towards creating the result you want.

Everything changed once I discovered there was such a thing as a cause towards a fitness objective. My entire approach towards getting in shape became incredibly straightforward and efficient. I was able to toss out 99% of the expensive and often trivial, rules governing how I should train or eat yet I would still make progress. As I learned more about root causes, I discovered some fascinating facts about them.

1. Root causes are the same for everyone

As I kept discovering bigger rocks, I noticed that the larger principles applied to people in a more uniform way. Once I hit on the cause, I was struck with the realization that at the root, we are all the same. It doesn't matter how young, old, rich, or poor you are. We are all the same at the root. We all lose weight, build muscle and become faster runners for the same root causes.

2. Root causes never change throughout your life

Underlying causes are like gravity. Despite the fact that jokes people make about how gravity affects the body as we age, the actual cause directing your results doesn't change over time. Root causes are universal natural principles that have been in place as long as there has been life on earth. They are the same today as they were yesterday and will continue until long after we're gone. They will always have the same power over you regardless of your life situation.

3. Every fitness goal has one, and only one, cause

This lesson made things simple. Once I learned what the cause of things like fat loss or body sculpting was I didn't feel the need to keep searching for something that would or wouldn't work. In a sense, I felt like I had figured out this whole fitness thing.

It took a few years to figure out what the most common root causes are, but once I knew what they were fitness was no longer a mystery to me. The only question became how I could fulfill the purpose, but outside of that I felt I had this whole fitness puzzle pretty much solved.

4. It doesn't matter how you fulfill the cause of your goal

Not only does the cause hold the key to the results you want, but it also gives you the freedom and flexibility to achieve those results however you wish. You don't have to abide by the rules of the latest diets. You also don't have to do exercises you don't enjoy or use equipment you don't want to use. If you're struggling to find motivation to stick to a certain workout, or worry about maintaining a particular method you're now free to ditch it and use something else that agrees with your lifestyle and preferences.

5. The cause is the most direct and quickest way to reach your goals

Root causes are the ultimate shortcut in fitness. I know, lots of experts like to take the stance that there are no shortcuts when it comes to getting in shape, but believe me, there are loads of shortcuts. I even would argue that you can't get in shape without them!

In fitness, a short cut is anything that makes it easier, and cheaper to do the necessary work to fulfill the cause of your goal. If a particular method means you can satisfy the same root cause but with less cost, then it's a short cut. If a workout takes you 60 minutes and costs $30, but you figure out how to do the same thing in 30 minutes for free then that's a short cut. You still have to do the work of fulfilling the cause, but that doesn't mean you always have to pay through the nose to do it.

6. The cause empowers you to gain better results

The shortest distance between two points is a straight line. The cause of your goal is that straight line between the point you're at now and the destination you want to reach. Fulfilling the cause means you can achieve the same results much more efficiently, but it also means you can go much further. It's just like discovering a 50% off sale. You have the option to save money, or you can get twice as much for the price you originally paid.

7. Many experts gloss over the root causes or even claim that they don't even matter in the first place

You may be asking yourself; if the cause is so powerful why doesn't every fitness expert in the world focus on it? The answer is because some experts either don't fully understand just how important they are while others even claim that the cause of things like fat loss or improving performance doesn't even exist. I've even been criticized for teaching people about them from folks claiming that I'm behind the times and not up on the latest "science."

When you consider how much modern dogmas decry the essential causes responsible for success its no surprise there's so many struggles to stay in shape. Over the years, I've noticed this sort of attitude more and more. The biggest reason why fitness can be such a struggle for so many people is that we place far too much emphasis on the things that aren't that important while essential principles are considered trivial. It's the classic example of being penny wise but pound foolish.

8. Root causes are from Mother Nature and mankind invented dogmas

Learning about the underlying causes was both liberating and humbling. Like all fitness enthusiasts, I have my bias and beliefs about what methods are best. The root causes have taught me that even though my favorite methods are effective, they were not that important. For example, I had always believed free weights were better than machines for building muscle, but now I realized that, for some goals, it doesn't matter if I lift with free weights, machines, springs, bands or just carried rocks around. It's the cause that is important, not the method used to fulfill it.

Each of the primary root causes is the most rock-solid law governing not just your body but the universe as a whole. They are not a new-age theory or trend nor are they a traditional dogma that's been passed down through many generations. They are as dependable and reliable as the very laws of physics.

The root is the route

To drive home the idea of what root causes are, the power they hold and how many in our fitness culture relate to them I would like to conclude this chapter with a little story.

Imagine a scenario where you're in a city, and you need to get back to your hotel. After wandering around you come to a small group of people at a bus stop who might look like they know the city. You walk up and say "excuse me, could you tell me how to get to the hotel on the beach?"

"You need to take a cab," says one of them.

"No, you should take the bus. I know that hotel always has lots of buses in front of it."
"I highly recommend driving a car. I'm sure that will get you there."

Then another person says "Are you crazy, my uncle drove a car for 30 years and has never been to that hotel!"

Then someone shows up with a newspaper and recommends a motorcycle. "This study shows that 35% of all people in that hotel ride bikes. Apparently riding a bike will be your best chance to get there." At that point, a couple of individuals start to a debate over which motorcycle would be best for you to use.

By now a crowd has gathered, and someone says "no the guy who says you should drive a car is right, but it should be a Honda. My sister drives a Honda and goes right past that hotel every day." Back and forth the opinions are flying, and the debate is heating up. Some folks offer their services and products all aimed at helping you discover what you should drive to get to the hotel.

Finally, you just take a stab and ask the first guy where you can get a Honda, preferably a black one because you've also heard that the color of the car is important for some reason. There just so happens to be a car dealership across the street. So you go across and buy a black Honda. Once behind the wheel, you're ready to get to your hotel. You head out of the parking lot and drive down the road. And you drive, and drive and drive. It's been hours, and you've had to stop and fill your tank with gas. And still, you continue to drive. At this point, one of two things can happen. You either do get to your hotel by chance, or you don't and give up.

Let's say you give up. You abandon your car by the side of the road, and you think "well that might have worked for someone else, but it didn't work for me. I guess I'm different." If someone asks you how to get to that hotel, you tell them "I wouldn't recommend a black Honda. Maybe that motorcycle theory had something to it, though."

Or let's say you do get to your hotel. After hours of driving around the city, you somehow stumble upon the hotel and think "hey it worked!" While at the hotel your friend calls you up and says you should get together for drinks. "No problem," You say. "Just drive around in a black Honda and you'll be here in a few hours, but make sure you have enough cash to buy another tank of gas."

I know this story might be kind of silly, but this is what happens every day within our fitness culture. People, who are seeking out a destination, pick a vehicle and just start going without any idea what the best route is. Every time someone recommends running for endurance, low carbohydrate diets for fat loss and balance disks for functional training they are doing the same thing as the folks recommending the Honda or taxi cab. They are recommending what vehicle you should use, but your chances of success never depend on upon just having a particular method and spending as much as you can to use it.

The cause of your goals is the actual path or road you need to travel. If you asked for directions, you would expect the person to say something like "Go 2 miles down Main Street and make a left onto Beech Street. It'll be on your left a couple of blocks up." Little to no mention of the vehicle would need to be said. Everyone would assume you would already have some method you can use.

But, ask most folks how to lose weight or build muscle and you'll hardly ever hear anything about the actual path you need to take. Instead, you'll receive lots of recommendation about what vehicles to use. You'll hear suggestions like how much cardio to do, what sorts of machines to work out on or what foods you should or shouldn't eat. While this might seem like good advice, it's not any different than asking for directions to a destination and being told you need to drive an individual vehicle.

Using different vehicles explains why some things might "work" for some people but not for others. The success of reaching a fitness goal is not about the vehicle but how well someone travels the most efficient path. If twenty people went up to the same street corner and asked to go to the same hotel, they would all receive the same set of directions. It doesn't matter how they were different from each other. They were all going to the same place, and the same route would get them all there.

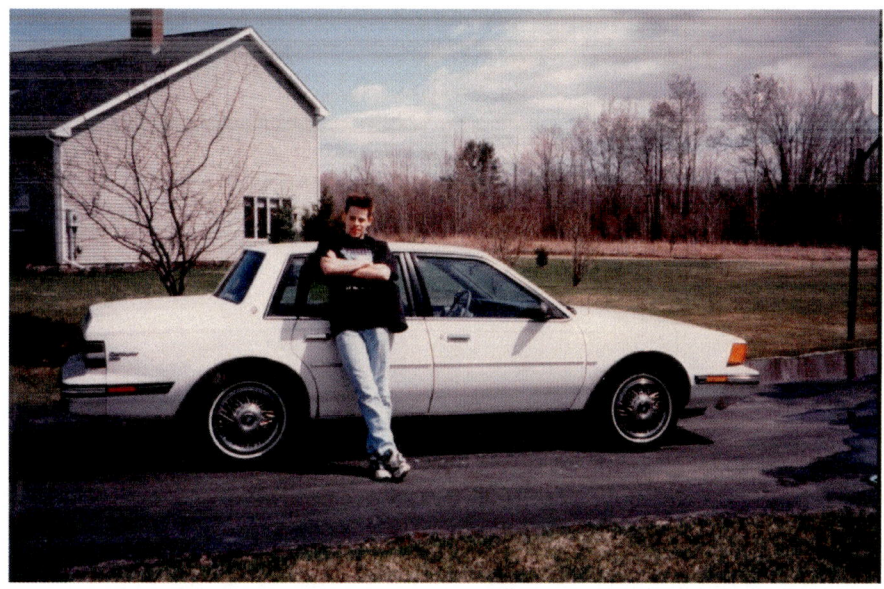

My first car at 17, and it got me around town just as well as a Rolls Royce as long as I didn't get lost.

Fitness Independence is about staying route, or root, focused. When you know the most direct path, you can pick whatever vehicle you like best. Maybe you prefer to ride a bike, or perhaps even walk. You might have a different car or truck. When your mind focuses on using the "right vehicle" you can spend untold amounts of lifestyle resources hopping from one car to the next and wasting, even more, resources using them. If you don't get to your destination, you believe the vehicle didn't work and discredit the value it can still bring you. If you do reach your goal you might feel you have to use that, and only that, method. In both cases, you are limited in both your freedom and potential to achieve results.

Once you know the cause, you can focus on traveling the most direct route with the resources you have and the methods you enjoy using. It's because of this you can do things your way, the way you want to do them and get better results through the easiest and most efficient means possible.

3: Surface Influences

When I started teaching folks to focus on root causes, I often got a lot of pushback and disbelief. "You mean I can lose weight, and it doesn't matter what I eat or how many meals I eat during the day?" "Surely you can't be serious that someone can get strong, but it doesn't matter what sort of program they are on!" And I would often get questions asking me things like "Okay, I get what you're saying, but what about this thing I read about in study X or magazine Y?"

I can understand why there is a lot of confusion out there. Our fitness culture has told folks for years, and built massive businesses, around that idea that you need to do 101 different things to achieve success. Now, here I am claiming that as long as you focus on just one or two simple things, everything else doesn't matter.

The truth is focusing on the cause doesn't mean everything else doesn't matter. In fact, it's just the opposite. Everything else *does* matter. Every tiny little seemingly insignificant thing matters. If you're baking cookies and lick the spoon, that single lick matters. If you take the stairs instead of the elevator, that single flight of stairs counts. Once you understand the cause of your goal, you'll learn that everything in your life matters regardless of what it is. However, while every single thing in your life does matter, none of these details are entirely in control of your results. Instead, they are influences to the cause of your goal. They play a part, but they are never responsible for the whole story. These details are what I call the surface influences.

In the analogy of getting to your hotel, the surface forces are the vehicles you consider or the condition of the road. The bus, the taxi or the Honda are all influences. The cost of the bus fare is an influence. Even the amount of gas in the car is an influence. Surface influences are just about anything and everything that can have some say towards your fitness habits. They can include anything from the friends you keep to the dog you walk each day.

Our fitness culture is obsessed with influences. Almost every book, study, blog post, and seminar is all about how some aspect of your lifestyle is influencing the causes of your fitness. The only problem is that these influences are not portrayed as a minor force but rather as a direct cause. Examples include how sports improve academic standing. How sugar can contribute to weight gain or how a particular type of exercise will improve muscle building. While there may be a link between playing sports to getting good grades, that doesn't mean that someone will earn high marks just because they run track. It doesn't say that eating a candy bar will always make you fatter.

Influential over reliance

When people become too focused on a particular influence, while ignoring the cause, their approach towards fitness become bent and distorted. Focusing too much on a particular detail is what I call influential over-reliance which is when someone believes all of their success rests on one or two limited influences. Examples may include when someone places all of their fat loss hopes on eating certain foods, or they believe they will build muscle if they use the right equipment or lift within a certain rep range.

Focusing too much on a single influence restricts your lifestyle flexibility while also limiting your potential for success. It causes you to rest your full weight on influence, which has limited power to produce results while making you blind to the plethora of other influences that can undermine or accelerate your progress.

Here are a few typical examples of influential over-reliance:

- Someone may be cutting out sugar in their diet to lose weight, but they are blind to the role other "safe or clean" foods can still play in making them gain weight.

- A middle age man believes running is the best way to stay lean, so he forces a harsh running schedule upon himself, all the while ignoring the role his diet and sleep habits play in his body fat levels.

- A young teen believes lifting free weights is the best way to build muscle. Because of this, he always makes sure he only uses free weights, all the while ignoring his lack of technical skill which is setting him up for injury and frustration.

- A recently retired gentleman decides to get interested in golf and spends a fortune on hiring a coach to perfect his swing. He practices every week for hours but ignores the fact that his tight and weak back is preventing him from lowering his handicap.

- A young football player believes a particular exercise is the absolute best way to train for his position. He dedicates a lot of his time to practicing this move and continues to do it even though he's experiencing pain from the exercise. Since it's "the best" he continues to force himself to do it until injury forces him off the field.

Over-reliance on influences can lock you into a prison of your design, but that doesn't mean you can, or should, ignore an influence. Just because I may be eating a chocolate chip cookie, and I say I'm not worried about weight gain, that doesn't mean I think that cookie has no influence to my body fat. All I'm saying is I can fit cookies into my diet and still keep the cause governing my body fat under control. That's the magic of understanding how surface influences relate to your root causes. To help further understand the relationship between the two here are a few comparison points to consider.

1. **Root causes are few; influences are practically infinite**

You can count on one hand the number of root causes within our fitness culture. In contrast, there are as many surface influences as there are grains of sand on a beach. Anything and everything can be an influence. Your friends, family, and coworkers can be an influence. Your car, the commute you drive and even the music you listen to can be an influence. Essentially anything that can alter your daily habits can be an impact towards your fitness goals.

2. Influences are different for everyone

While root causes are universal, influences are different for everyone. The only way someone will have the same influences as you are if they have the same life you do. The same job, the same friends, even the same genetics. So unless you have a twin who is living your same life, then your influences are as unique to you as your fingerprints.
These details are where that whole "different things work for different people" comes into play. Your influences affect how much various fitness habits affect your outcome. If you and a friend go on the same diet, but experience different results, it doesn't mean that you're different when it comes to getting in shape. It means you both have unique influences that slightly alter how well that diet fulfilled the cause of your goal.

3. Influences are always changing

Once again, root causes are the same, and they stay the same. Influences, on the other hand, can change day by day and even minute by minute.

Take for example the food in your fridge. The foods you have in your environment will profoundly influence your diet. I'm willing to bet that the food choices you have in your fridge will be different tomorrow than they are right now. You'll have more of some foods, not much of another and maybe too much of something else. If someone brings cookies into the office, your nutritional influences shift. They would also change in a different way if they brought in the fruit salad.

4. Trying to control influences can be stressful and exhausting

Trying to control your fitness through tightly controlling your influences is no different than trying to control life itself. Your influences are in a constant state of change, and most of them are completely out of your control. Sure, you might be able to stock your fridge with the foods you like, but the menu during a power lunch may be a different story.

Proper planning will help, but you can't control everything and trying to do so will undoubtedly cause lots of stress. Worrying about every detail is one of the primary reasons why fitness can be very stressful for so many people. By focusing on the cause of your goals, you can take stock of the influences that are easiest to control and let life do its thing without worrying too much about it.

5. Experts often place far too much importance on various influences

Unlike root causes, Influences all have limited weight in how much they can help you. There isn't influence that is 100% responsible towards your goals. Sugar or red meat isn't wholly responsible for weight gain. Running can't directly cause fat loss. Organic food doesn't guarantee a healthy diet and doing bicep curls doesn't promise anyone bigger biceps. You wouldn't know it from much of the fitness literature. Pick up any diet book or hit a bodybuilding website and you'll quickly come under the impression that biceps curls will jack up your arms, sugar will make you fat, and running will make you shed pounds.

Once I came to understand the importance of causes and the limited power of influences it made complete sense as to why the failure rate within our fitness culture was so high. Every year lots of people pile influences into their lives hoping to get what they want yet they fall short. The firm focus on little details is one of the biggest reasons why so many people spend lifestyle resources and never get what they want. It's entirely possible to focus on a few diet and exercise influences and still never fulfill the cause of the goal. Your success depends 100% on how well you fulfill the cause, not how well you control a handful of influences.

6. Big influences usually have high lifestyle costs

Some influences are massive and can make a huge dent towards fulfilling your cause. The only problem is those big influences sometimes have large lifestyle costs. Spending too much on a few select influences is a big reason why some folks spend themselves into a dead end or plateau. They keep trying to maximize a few key influences until they can't use any more time and energy. They've maxed out their resources yet are nowhere close to where they want to be because that influence is limited in how well it can fulfill the cause. While they have maxed out their potential to control a few influences, there are other influences they are not paying attention to that can sabotage their ability to fulfill the cause of their goal.

A typical example of this is the person who's trying to lose or maintain weight entirely through cardio based exercise. To keep burning more fat or calories, they have to spend more time and energy working out. Eventually, they are at their limit of how much they are willing to exercise, and they hit a dead end. In their mind, they are doing everything right, but they are ignoring other influences to their weight such as dietary choices and lifestyle habits that can wipe out the fat loss influences of the exhausting workouts.

7. Influences are bigger for some folks and smaller for others

The same influence might be big for you but relatively minor for someone else. For example, say you and a friend both swear off drinking for a month. Unless you both drink the same amount of the same drinks the influence of drinking will be different for both of you. If you drink one beer a week, and your friend drinks three beers a day then giving up beer will be a much bigger influence on your friend than for you.

The same example applies towards exercise. If you run 20 miles a week, and your friend never goes running, then going for a jog during lunch time will be a much bigger influence on your friend than for yourself. Again, this can contribute to the idea that different things work for different people. It's not that we are different in how we become fit, it's because we all have different influences.

Influences can work more for you at one point in your life than at another. You may have lost thirty pounds on a particular diet when you were back in college, but for some reason, you only lost five pounds fifteen years later. Most of it has to do with how much the rules of that diet were an influence. The rules of the diet were a bigger influence when you were younger, and now the influence diminished due to various other lifestyle factors.

8. Surface Influences are powerful in numbers but often weak by themselves

Most influences are pretty minor. The appliances in your kitchen are an influence towards your diet. If you suddenly gain or lose a new cooking tool, it's a safe bet that your diet won't change much. Even the condition of your walking shoes can play a role. If your shoes are worn out, you may not want to go for a walk. So while you could argue that good shoes or a new slow cooker might improve your health, they are a drop in the bucket compared to all of the other influences that remain the same. The limited power of surface influences is why you can make a few small changes in your life, yet not experience much in the way of results.

9. Influences are often to blame for genetics, set points and "the way we are"

There are a lot of ideas within our fitness culture which suggest that it's tough to make personal changes in fitness. Some people blame genetics, and others point to a set point theory where your body naturally adjusts towards the same condition. I've even heard some people say they can't change because "that's just the way they are." Most of the time, this tendency to stay the same is due to maintaining the same influences. People are creatures of habit so our daily routine is pretty consistent and therefore so are our daily influences. When your influences experience little change, your habits stay pretty much the same and thus so do the fulfillment of the root causes.

If you experience a dramatic shift in your lifestyle, like moving away to college, working a new job, adding a new member to the family or even going on a vacation your daily influences can change on mass. When these events occur, change seems much more inevitable. In many cases, it can be difficult *not* to change your level of fitness.
The power of many influences does not mean you need to move or go back to school to change, but it's a good example of why the bulk of your daily influences can prevent you from making much headway even though you're doing your best to change what you can.

Some common influences

While there can be an infinite number of influences towards any goal here are some of the biggest ones you can focus on towards fulfilling the cause.

1. **Objectives and goals**

Your goals are the initial spark that makes everything else happen in your fitness lifestyle. It's a destination which influences every choice and action you make from here on out. Without knowing what you want, every decision you make is going to be a random guess at best. The clearer you are on what you want the more efficient your choices can become. You'll know what programs and products are going to be a waste of your resources and which ones will be well worth your investment.

2. **Preferences and resources**

Many experts will tell you that the best diet or workout program is the one you're willing to stick to and the program you'll stick to are probably the one you enjoy. It doesn't matter if running is great for fat loss or if you should give up chocolate. If you really don't want to do either of those things, chances are you won't maintain those habits. Understanding the cause of your goal gives you the freedom to pick whatever methods so you can pick and choose the influences you employ or ignore.

When it comes to your resources, you can't use what you don't have. It's hard to implement a plan that requires 3 hours a day of training time when you can hardly spare 20 minutes. I once had a goat farmer in Pakistan ask me how to get stronger even though the closest gym was several hours away. It would have been crazy to me to suggest an equipment intensive strength program. Instead, we used resources he had on hand including hills, rocks, logs, a cart and even the goats themselves.

3. **Your energy level**

Your energy level is a massive influence towards almost every fitness goal possible. You must have the physical and emotional fuel to do the work necessary to fulfill the cause of your goal. When your energy level is high, even the hardest work seems easier. When it's low, it can be almost impossible to do the smallest tasks. Don't get caught up in the idea that being tired and burning the candle at both ends is a sign of a strong work ethic. You'll only spend your energy wisely if you can use it productively which is in the fulfillment of your cause.

4. **Sleep**

Your sleep routine holds a massive influence on your energy level and thus everything you want to accomplish. Poor sleep habits do nothing more than slow your progress to a crawl. They don't make you tougher or stronger. It's just the opposite. Many of our fitness problems boil down to a lack of sleep, and many "solutions" try to make up for the effects of lack of rest. Get a good night's sleep as consistently as possible and everything you want to accomplish will become much easier.

5. Diet and nutrition

I cover diet and nutrition in a separate chapter, but it's worth noting what you eat is a pretty significant influence in everything you do. Much of this is because your diet is a major influence towards your energy level. While the amount of power food can vary from goal to goal, it's seldom ever a minor impact.

6. Friends and family

Never underestimate the influence of the people closest to you. They are some of, if not the most influential voices in your life. A lot of folks blame the media and the Internet when it comes to fitness expectations. While the media is a fitness influence, it's practically powerless compared to your friends and family. If your parents were strong chances are their influence spilled over into your life. Spending a ski weekend with your family is a much bigger impact than any commercial or magazine ad for a ski vacation.

Your friends also influence your choices. Chances are, your habits and attitudes are going to be much more like your friends than anyone else. The social pull of friends can also grow with age. At the age of 38, I can confidently say the majority of my fitness habits came about because of what my friends did at some point in my life.

7. Mentors, coaches, and teachers

Every lesson you learn, be it from a book, a seminar or just a talk over coffee is one of the biggest influences towards your habits from that moment forth. It's for this reason that you must pick and choose your teachers wisely. They not only guide you but teach you based on what they believe. Some of these beliefs may serve you well, others maybe not. One of my first coaches once said to me "Matt, I'm giving you the best information I've got. Your job is to figure out what is useful to you and what advice you should discard."

8. Your environment

Your environment is a massive influence in your daily lifestyle and fitness. This includes everything from the climate to what sort of terrain you encounter. There's a good reason why some of the best winter athletes come from parts of the world that include both snow and mountains. You'll be hard pressed to find an Olympic downhill skier who grew up in Kansas, but there are more than a few from Northern California and Colorado.

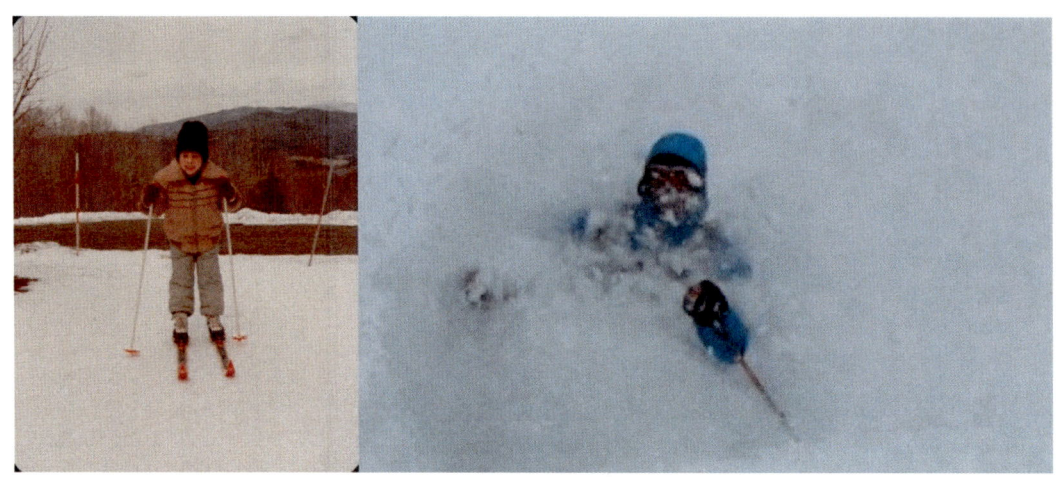

Snow has always been a big influence in my life.

Don't let your current environment discourage you. All environments offer many opportunities to be active and healthy. Maybe you live near a lake you can swim in. If not, maybe there's a bike path nearby. There's always something useful right around the corner.

9. What you believe and know

Lastly, everything you do is heavily influenced by what you know and feel to be true about the world. Human history is written based upon people's beliefs. The very fact that you are reading this book is the result of a series of beliefs you've adopted over time.

Keep in mind that personal development and growth often involves challenging ideas you've held onto for many years. The more your feelings stay the same, the more your actions and habits will stay the same. It doesn't matter if your ideas are right or wrong. If they never change, you'll never change.

The human ego is stubborn. People have been killed, enslaved, impoverished and had their lives ruined because of their beliefs. The purpose of this book isn't to tell you what's right or wrong but rather to present you with a set of beliefs I've adopted and have served me well. Your job is to take them in and let them digest for a while. Your mind uses information just as your body uses food. It will break things down and decide what to do with what it's consumed. Only then will you be able to figure out what is best for you and what you should discard.

All surface influences are important, but none of them are in control of your results. Trying to gain full control of your influences is not only incredibly stressful and impractical, but it's also not very effective. No matter how great your diet is or how hard you exercise your efforts will always have a limited effect. You don't have to pull your hair out because some influences work against you. You can just flow through life knowing that as long as you fulfill the cause, you'll be okay. Later on, I'll be exploring some sound strategies on how you can manipulate them to your advantage. Right now though let's cut right to the chase and start exploring the root causes of some of the most sought after fitness goals within our fitness culture.

Part II: Basic Principles

4: The Cause of Body Fat

Okay, you've got a handle on the cost of fitness, what root causes are and how they are different from the surface influences in your life. Now let's get your hands dirty and begin with one of the most sought after goals in fitness, fat loss.

Getting rid of and controlling how much fat is in the human body may be the single biggest motivating factor behind most of society's fitness habits. Sure, staying strong and living well are important, but imagine what would happen if people never had to worry about weight gain? I guess that long row of cardio equipment at your local gym would become a lot less popular. The demand for many of the supplements and diet foods would dry up overnight.

The ultimate fat loss goal isn't fat loss

I once heard a wealthy philosopher say that one of the best things someone can do is to "get the whole money thing out of the way." Try to get yourself in a financial position where you don't have to spend the majority of your lifestyle resources paying the bills and putting food on the table. Otherwise, you'll compromise your ability to help both yourself and the world around you when you spend most of your energy just keeping your head above water financially.

I have spent far too many years working my tail off just to get by. Only instead of working to pay the bills, I was spending most of my resources just to manage the fat levels on my body. Weight management can be a huge drain on lifestyle resources. It's so massive that the primary focus for many diet and exercise programs is all about getting and staying lean. There was a time when I believed this obsession was a good thing, but not anymore. Basing your eating habits and exercise plans on weight management alone is akin to spending all of your time and energy working just to pay the bills. It's not a bad thing, but you're merely getting by while there is a whole world of fantastic experiences you're too busy to experience. A healthy lifestyle can be, and should be much more than just keeping a lean physique.

So get the whole fat loss thing taken care of and out of the way as soon as possible. If you want to lose weight, get it off and be done with it. Fat loss shouldn't be a lifelong journey. It's like driving cross country. Get started, get to your destination and continue with your life. There's nothing that says you have to spend your life focused on battling the bulge. Life is much better when there's one less thing you have to worry about on a daily basis. Our fitness culture loves to portray an image where those who are the most disciplined about their weight enjoy the spoils of life. I used to think that way too, but now I see things differently. Food tastes much better when you don't concern yourself with counting calories or looking up how much sugar is in a cookie. Physical activity is a heck of a lot more fun when you're not always focusing on staying in a fat burning zone on your heart rate monitor.

You may be thinking that such a carefree approach towards weight management may not be possible for you, that it's a pipe dream only the top 1% might reach after years of effort. I promise you this objective is not out of reach. I believe it's a state anyone can achieve, and the first step is in understanding what body fat is, and the cause that changes how much of it is on your body.

Where does fat come from?

If you asked most people where the fat on their body comes from they might say it comes from sugar, cupcakes, or fried and processed foods. I can't deny that something like fried butter at the country fair is an influence, but the origin of fat goes back much further than what is on your plate. In fact, the ultimate source of your body fat doesn't even originate on this planet. The journey of your body fat begins from a source that's about 93 million miles away. It comes from that great big atom smashing nuclear fusion reactor known as the sun.

All energy on Earth originates from the sun including the very fat you're carrying around right now. I know that might seem a little strange. It's not like you can get fat by stepping outside on a sunny day. That's because we humans lack the capacity to directly harness the sun's energy for sustenance. Luckily we have a helping hand from plants and vegetation.

Plants take in the sun's energy, and through photosynthesis, can bind carbon (from the carbon dioxide in the air) and hydrogen (from water) atoms together like this:

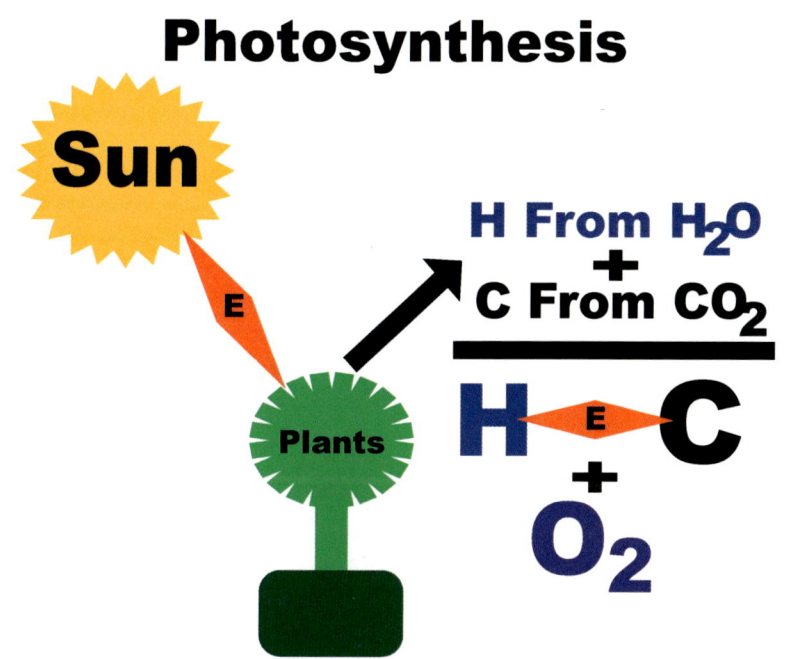

Energy comes from the sun, and is stored in the bond between hydrogen from water and carbon from carbon dioxide with Oxygen as a waste product.

What you're looking at here is the magical source of fuel for us humans. This bond between carbon and hydrogen is the energy we gain through ingesting those plants in the form of simple sugars and fiber. So while we may not be able to harness the energy of the sun directly, plants serve as a middleman to package that energy through photosynthesis so we can consume and utilize it.

The Human Fuel Cell

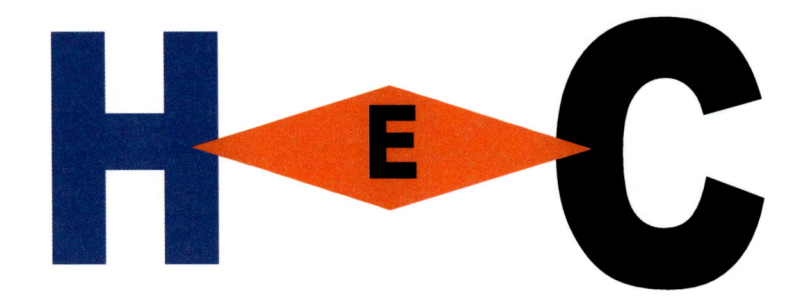

H — E — C

The energy you live off of comes from the energy stored in the bond between hydrogen and carbon, the product of photosynthesis.

Also, animals consume those plants and create protein and fat by using those same carbon and hydrogen bonds as the primary building blocks. You then consume those animals and in turn consume the energy they have ingested from plants.

The energy you use to survive and run your physical systems exists in this *chemical bond,* and you can take it into our body through any food or beverage source you like. You can even take it in intravenously. It's in everything from organic vegetables to deep fried hot dogs. The primary difference between that hot dog and some organic carrots is the concentration of how many carbon and hydrogen bonds in each bite. The hot dog probably has many more of those bonds in a single bite than in a handful of carrots.

Of course, it can be tricky to tell how many carbon and hydrogen bonds there are in a given food. There can be millions or even billions of them. To simplify the ability to track how much energy food has we use the term "calorie."

The mysterious calorie

The calorie is one of the most misunderstood concepts within our fitness culture. One of the biggest misconceptions is that food is calories and calories are food. A typical example of this is when people talk about protein calories and how they are different from carbohydrate calories and so on. The key is to understand that we gain calories *from* fat, protein, and carbohydrates. These macronutrients are not calories in and of themselves.

When you need to use the energy from photosynthesis you don't directly use those atoms or the physical substance that is food. The energy is of that bond, not the atoms (aka the foodstuffs) themselves. Once you use that energy, you have a carbon atom and a hydrogen atom just floating around kind of like discarded pizza boxes in a college dorm room. They are essentially a waste product. If those hydrogen and carbon atoms build up, your body will become one heck of a toxic environment.

Thankfully, you take in oxygen through the air you breathe. You combine that carbon to 2 Oxygen atoms and breathe it out in the form of CO2. You also combine that hydrogen atom to the oxygen and expel it as H2O or water in your breath, sweat, and urine.

The cause of fat level changes

The root of how much fat is on your body is quite simple. What you have is a given container or amount of space (your body) and a given amount of something (fat aka. energy) within that container. A change in the level of something within a space is the result of the cause of IN vs. OUT.

- How much money is in your bank account?
- How many cars are in the parking lot?
- How many people are in the room?
- How much water is in the lake?
- How many stars are in the galaxy?
- How much fat is in your body?

The answer to all of these questions boils down to the balance between the speeds at which how much is going into that space against the speed it's going out. If more of a substance is going in a space than is going out the level of that thing will rise. If more goes out of the space than is going in the level will drop. If the amount going out is the same as the amount going in, then the level will remain the same.

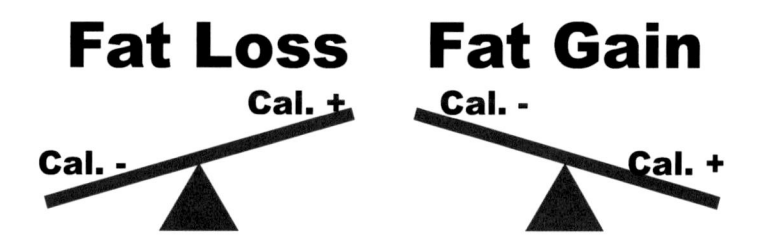

Fat Loss   Fat Gain
Cal. +   Cal. -
Cal. -   Cal. +

Fat Maintenance
Cal. -   Cal. +

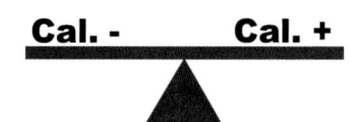

Losing or gaining fat isn't about diet or exercise alone, but the balance between calorie intake and expenditure.

The most important thing to understand is that it's the *balance* between the rates you have calories going in vs., the rate calories are going out. The individual numbers of calorie intake or expenditure are not ultimately in control. Having a million dollars go into your bank account with a million going out will give you the same bank statement as someone who hasn't made a penny. It's not about the intake or the expenditure, but the *balance* between the two.

Understanding the balance of intake and expenditure is essential to achieving both fat loss and Fitness Independence. When you expend more caloric energy than you consume your body fat level drops. If you consume more caloric energy than you're expending, you will gain body fat. If the level is the same on both sides, your body fat levels will stay the same.

I know, it's simple, but I feel it's important to hammer home this point because many theories dispute the fact that the amount of fat on your body is all about the speed of calories in vs. calories out. Far too many plans you fat loss through a particular diet or exercise "trick." While such a trick can be an *influence* towards your calorie balance, no single diet or exercise method can ever be fully in controlling your fat levels and guarantee a lean physique. What most folks perceive as a cause is an influence that can alter the calorie balance by chance. To understand why to let's look at the details about how you can change that all important calorie balance.

The intake half of the calorie and fat balance

From an energy perspective, the fat on your body isn't much different than the fat, protein and carbohydrate in your diet. It's a battery for the life fueling energy between those carbon and hydrogen atoms. The cause doesn't care what nutrition battery you consume. The energy in fat, protein, and carbohydrates is the same. A lot of folks claim there is a difference between fat calories or carbohydrate calories and so on. It's true that the body uses fat, protein, and carbohydrates in different influential ways, but the actual calories contained in those nutrients is the same. They all come from the same source which is the sun. The only way you can consume different types of calories is if you start consuming foods grown under a different sun.

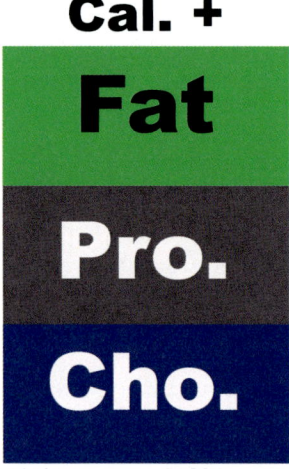

Your calorie intake (cal.+) is composed of fat, protein and carbohydrate.

Anything you eat, drink or consume with fat, protein, and carbohydrate will be an influence to the intake half of your caloric balance. Your body is designed to take any form of calories and turn it into fat for storage. Body fat can come from any food you eat under any dietary conditions. There is no such thing as a source of calories that cannot influence your fat stores. *Note: I didn't include the possible fourth source of calories which is alcohol. If you consume alcoholic beverages, add those to the total calorie intake.

Of course, there's no guarantee the calories you consume will turn to fat, and even if they do, that's no guarantee your body fat levels will increase. It all depends on upon how your energy intake is balanced out by how much energy you are expending. The expenditure half of the calories balance is a lot more diverse than the intake half. Calories can exit your body in one of three ways:

1. Some calories can pass right through your digestive tract. It's as simple as in one end and out the other.
2. You can store calories in various ways. You can save calories in your fat, protein and carbohydrate storage tanks. If they are stored as fat, your fat levels *might* increase. If they are stored (or maybe used) as muscle or glycogen and blood sugar they will not.
3. Lastly, calories can be used to fuel your body.

Burning calories is the primary way your body expends the caloric energy consumed through food. While you can burn more energy in many different ways, all forms of caloric expenditure fall into one of three categories.

The three ways you burn calories

There are three ways you can use the calories that are not passed and remain in your body.

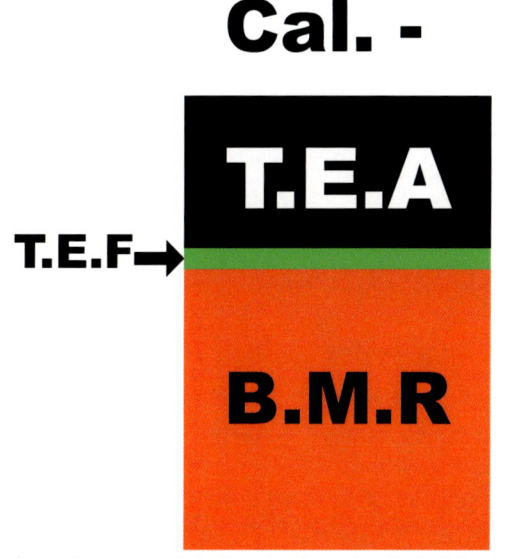

Calorie expenditure is composed of your base m metabolic rate, thermic effect of food and the thermic effect of activity.

1. **B.M.R**

B.M.R is your base metabolic rate and it's usually the biggest influence towards your caloric expenditure. It's the energy you spend to keep your body doing what it does even if you're just lying in bed.

Unfortunately, there's not much you can do to make large changes to your BMR. Most of the significant influences are out of your control. These include age, gender, general build, height, genetics and so on. There are a few smaller influences you can change like how much lean body mass you have. However, even with that, it's difficult to make large changes happen. Some folks can make a significant change to their BMR due to massive lifestyle changes, but these examples are outliers that are experiencing far more stress than the average fitness enthusiast.

2. **Thermic Effect of Food (T.E.F.)**

The Thermic Effect of Food is the energy you use to consume and digest the foods you eat. T.E.F. is a relatively small influence to the expenditure half of the calorie balance. Of course, that depends on how much food you eat and, to a certain extent, what you eat as well. The more food you take in, the more your body needs to work to process that food. Some foods require more work by your body to break down than others. Some diet plans rest their fat shedding laurels on this influence, but it's not always the most efficient plan. While a steak may require more energy to digest compared to a piece of chocolate, it's only a minor influence toward your T.E.F which is a small impact on the total amount of calories burned which is only half of the calorie balance equation.

Have the steak because you want steak, not because it means you'll burn a few extra calories. Plus, don't forget you have to consume calories to increase your T.E.F. You might spend an extra 20 calories digesting the steak, but it means eating an extra 300 calories worth of steak to do it so you're still in a net gain.

Some theories propose that various foods may require more calories to digest than the food itself supplies. If you eat 50 calories worth of carrots but it takes your body 60 calories to digest them then you've created a ten calorie deficient. There is some debate over if this is true but it's a safe bet that it's a pretty small influence to your total calorie balance. You would probably need to stick to a pretty extreme diet to make your T.E.F a large impact on your total caloric expenditure.

3. **Thermic Effect of Activity. (T.E.A.)**

The thermic effect of activity is the saving grace in your quest to burn fat and calories. While it's difficult to substantially change your BMR and T.E.F, you can change your T.E.A. considerably at any time. You can burn anywhere from a few hundred calories a day to thousands of calories a day just by changing your T.E.A.

The cool thing about T.E.A. is that it refers to all activity you do. It's not limited to exercise or to working out in a gym. Just standing up and walking around will boost your T.E.A. Everything you do with your body will count towards your calorie expenditure regardless of what you're doing and how you do it. It's liberating to know that all physical activity burns calories when popular fat loss methods emphasize hard exercise. All calories are equal regardless of how you burn them off. Ten calories burned playing with the dog has the same fat burning influence as burning ten calories while struggling through a workout.

The 3 Components of T.E.A

Just as you can break the expenditure half of the calorie balance into three categories (B.M.R, T.E.F, and T.E.A) you can also break the up the influences of T.E.A. into three categories. Whenever you want to burn more calories, all you need to remember is muscle, time and intensity.

Increasing Cal. -

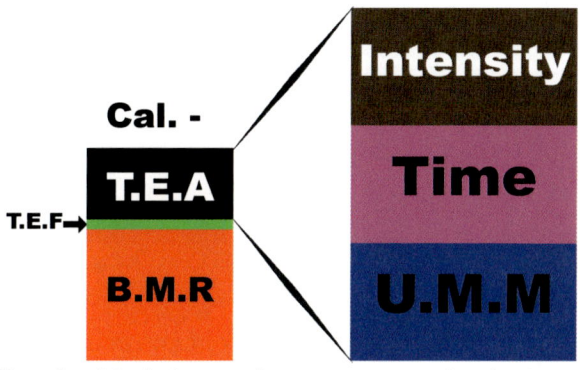

You can increase your thermic effect of activity by how much you use your muscles, the time you use them for and the intensity of the activity you do.

1. **UMM stands for Use More Muscle**

The more muscle you engage in an activity, the more calories you expend. Climbing a flight of stairs uses the large muscles in your legs which are why that activity burns more energy than say, opening and closing your hand as fast as you can around a squeeze ball.

Using more muscle is also why some of the best calorie burning exercises involve as much of the body as possible. Examples include swimming, X-C skiing, kickboxing, wrestling, full-body weightlifting exercises and so on.

2. **Intensity**

Increasing the intensity of activity will increase the amount of energy you spend per unit of time. You can do this by moving faster, like running instead of walking, or add resistance like lifting more weight, or crank up the resistance on a stationary bike.

3. Time

The longer you do something, the more calories you burn. Running for twenty minutes burns more calories than running for ten but not as much as running for thirty.

These are the three influences that govern T.E.A., and you can manipulate them for any form of exercise or activity. There's no need to debate over which exercises are best for fat loss. You can adjust the variables of muscle, intensity and time to alter the calorie burn for anything you like. It also puts to rest the idea that some exercises are best for fat loss. All exercises can potentially burn a lot of calories while all exercises can burn very few depending on how much that exercise can increase your T.E.A.

So that's the long and the short of it how you can change your body fat levels. Every ounce of fat you're holding right now comes down to the balance between calorie intake and calorie expenditure. Calories intake is influenced by the fat, protein, and carbohydrates you consume through food and drink. Calorie expenditure is influenced by T.E.A, BMR, and T.E.F, and T.E.A. is influenced by muscle use, intensity and time.

Lessons learned from the cause of calorie balance

Understanding how the influences of calorie balance impact the fat levels of your body brings some empowering and liberating notions to light.

The first lesson is that everything in your life, from your commute to what floor you live on can have a hand in how many calories you consume and expend. Nothing is immune and powerless. Even the size and cleanliness of your kitchen can play a role. If your kitchen is clean, you're more likely to use your kitchen to prepare a healthy meal, but coming home to a messy kitchen could be enough to temp you call out for pizza.

Expanding your awareness of your personal caloric influences is critical. Our fitness culture tends to create a focused view on what influences are most important when it comes to your fat levels. Some claim you should focus on sugar or fat. Other experts recommend focusing on your heart rate during a particular type of exercise like running. While these influences are important, don't make the mistake of becoming too focused on them. Obsessing over small details can cause you to ignore other influences that may matter just as much, maybe even more, and can sabotage your fat loss efforts.

The second and the more interesting lesson is that the level of fat on your body is entirely dependent upon the *balance* between how many calories you burn vs., how many you consume. While anything and everything can influence this balance nothing has direct and absolute control over it. The lack of control means there is no such thing as food, diet, exercise, workout, or supplement that can control your body fat levels.

Running 5 miles a day is only an *influence* towards your T.E.A., and that's just an influence towards the expenditure half of your total calories balance. So running those 5 miles can't possibly guarantee that you'll lose weight or stay lean. It's just an influence of an influence after all.

The same idea may apply to eating a particular food, like a slice of pizza. The energy in that slice is merely an influence of the intake half of the balance. It doesn't have the power to ensure you'll get fatter. Nothing you eat, by itself, can ever directly cause fat loss simply because of its chemical or nutritional makeup. Some foods may have more influence than others, but eating a slice of cake after dinner can't guarantee weight gain any more than a protein shake you consume after a workout.

There are some ways you can take this information. On one hand, it means that you shouldn't rest your hopes of a leaner physique on the latest exercise trend or that article about "super foods that fight fat." On the other hand, it means you have all of the options in the world at your disposal. You can manage your body fat however you like. If you don't like doing cardio, you don't have to do it. If you don't like choking down protein shakes every morning you can give that up too. It also means you can eat foods you like and do activities you enjoy while still staying lean. Understanding that nothing has the direct power to make you thinner or fatter is an excellent thing. It means the power isn't in the food in your fridge or that heart rate based cardio program. It means the power is finally in your hands, and you can wield it however you wish.

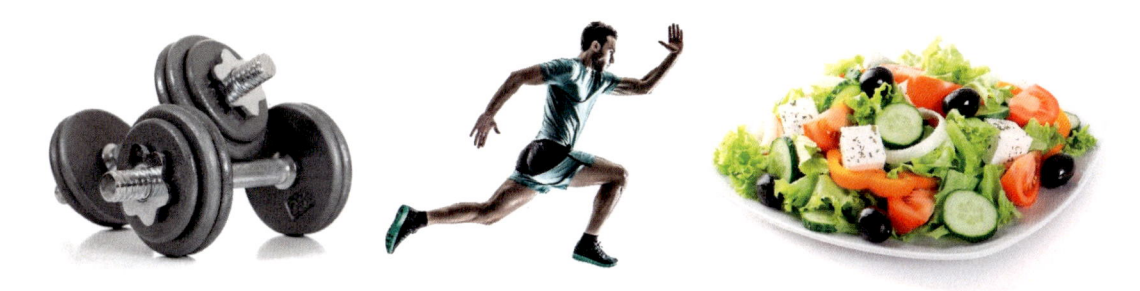

Our fitness culture blames many things for fat loss, but most of them are merely influences.

Now at this point, I only half expect the previous lessons to have the same empowering and liberating effect they had on me. After all, I learned all of this over the course of many years so I could learn and understand it gradually one step at a time. It took me a long while to eat a chocolate chip cookie and understand it couldn't make me any fatter all by itself. It took even longer to learn that I didn't have to do cardio to stay lean. I spent years believing a strict diet and the right workout program was essential. It took quite a while until I was able to let go of those ideas I was clinging to in fear that giving them up would cause weight gain.

I've also had the advantage to evaluate almost every objection to the notion of calorie balance and realize that none of them hold much water. You, on the other hand, are in the unfortunate situation of having me dump all of this on you in a few short moments. It can be a lot to take in, and there is an entire fitness culture out there telling you that "it's not that simple" or the media has discovered a new slimming workout and fat fighting food every month. It's because of this I would like to explore a few of the common arguments against calorie balance.

All calories are the same, but all foods are not

One of the biggest challenges for the cause of energy balance is the idea that all calories are not equal. That a fat calorie is different from a sugar calorie and so on.

The hiccup with this logic is in missing the fact that food and calories are not one and the same. To say calories are food is like saying batteries are electricity. Foods *contain* energy, but they are not the energy you use. While the food itself is different, calories are not. Various foods are different influences in your calorie balance. The corn dog you eat for lunch may have the same calories as a salad, but how these foods will influence your calorie balance may be different. The corn dog may not be as satisfying as the salad since the salad may take up more volume in your stomach, so you're not as likely to eat as much later throughout the day. So even though the caloric influences are the same, the food's impact towards your hunger or appetite may be different. Then again, we could debate that the fat and protein in the corn dog might make you feel more satisfied longer while the salad had little fat or protein so it might leave you feeling hungry 20 minutes later and craving the candy bar in the vending machine. We can debate the influence of the salad vs. the corn dog many ways, but most of them are just a distraction from what matters most which is the calorie balance.

No one ever got fatter by storing fat

Many diet and exercise methods like to focus on a particular aspect of science that says individual fitness habits cause fat to go in or out of your fat cells. Sometimes this has to do with hormones or a particular enzyme. Other times it may deal with heart rate zones or workout conditions like working out on an empty stomach. There is no shortage of theories. The tricky thing about these theories is they are mostly correct. Certain habits may shuttle fat to your fat cells and yes specific workout methods might suck fat right out of your fat cells like a vacuum cleaner. While these methods might seem scary or promising, they usually don't mean much overall.

The first reason is that you're always going to have fat going into your fat cells no matter what you do. The only way you can prevent fat from going into your fat cells is to never to consume any calories. Fat cells are there to store excess energy, so you have that energy to use during times when you're not eating. If you couldn't store fat, you would have a much harder time maintaining your health. Calorie storage gives you the freedom to live without always needing to eat or worry about your energy levels.

The second reason is that there's always more to the story than the single hormone or workout method to the energy balance. The fat on your body can go into, and come from, your fat cells along different routes. Trying to control or maximize one of those routes is no guarantee of success. It would be like trying to keep people from entering or leaving a football stadium and only controlling one exit. There are always many ways to gain and lose fat. If you focus on just one or two of those exits, you're missing out on the influential power of the others.

The third reason not to worry is that no one ever got fatter because fat went into their fat cells in the first place! Remember, we're dealing with a cause of calories coming in *and* calories being burned off. It's the balance between the amount of fat going into your fat cells vs. the fat going out that causes fat gain or loss. It really doesn't matter how much fat is going in or coming out of your fat cells.

Fat loss is about accelerating or slowing down something that's already happening

The super cool thing about the calorie balance is that you already have a steady flow of both caloric intake and caloric expenditure. Any fat loss strategy you adopt is about adjusting the speed of your intake and expenditure. It's not about starting or stopping some physiological process.

A typical example is when people talk about burning fat as if it only happens under a particular set of circumstance like eating the right foods or exercising the right way. Sometimes a supplement company will advertise that their product will "unlock" the fat in your cells and start burning it. All of these claims are untrue. You can't "start to burn fat" any more than you can begin to make the world spin. You're always burning and storing fat. It's a constant ongoing process that happens every single day. You don't have to start or stop doing anything to gain or lose body fat. You simply have to speed up or slow down the rate at which you consume and expend calories. Understanding the rate at which you consume and burn calories can be helpful if you want to build a plan for fat loss. You don't need to do anything special or crazy. All you need is to increase or decrease a few key habits you already have.

Calorie balance is not necessarily calorie counting

Another challenge I hear is from folks claiming they "did the whole calorie counting thing" and didn't lose weight. Therefore, it's not about a calorie balance and must be about something else. I wholeheartedly agree that calorie counting failed them, but that doesn't mean the cause of calorie balance isn't true.

Calorie counting can be a very hard and expensive undertaking. Most of the time, it is educated guessing at best. It's difficult because you need to have accurate numbers for both the calorie intake and calorie expenditure every day. If you get either side of the balance incorrect, you risk misunderstanding what's happening. So you aren't just trying to get one reading right, but two. Humans are notoriously bad at estimating anything having to do with size and quantity. Couple that with a poor memory and we're not exactly the best-suited machines for calorie counting. After all, what did you have for dinner last night? How much did each food weigh? Did you eat every bite of those foods? Personally, I can hardly remember what I ate 20 minutes ago let alone how many slices of turkey I had on that sandwich.

The good news is that calorie counting has become more accurate with advances in technology. Wearable electronic devices can help you track calorie expenditure through heart rate, body heat, and general movement. While these tools improve your accuracy, tracking caloric intake is still quite difficult. To accurately track every calorie, you need to account for every gram of food and every drop of drink. This means calorie counting has a high cost to accuracy ratio. The more accurate you're counting; the more lifestyle resources it will cost you.

I had a friend in college who was a master calorie counter. The downside was it cost her a lot every day. She refused to eat anything she couldn't buy, prepare and weigh on a scale for herself. Her high maintenance eating style meant she didn't eat out, and she had to bring her food to events like birthday parties and barbecues. She also had a strict routine when it came to tracking her energy expenditure. She had a super strict schedule for when she was to go to sleep and wake up in the morning. She measured her steps and even took note of how many times she climbed the three flights of stairs to her dorm room.

As you can imagine, this sort of lifestyle wasn't the easiest to maintain during the hectic years of her college career. Life is hard enough to wrestle into control, let alone trying to do it when every day has a different routine.

Calorie counting isn't
1+2=3
It's more like

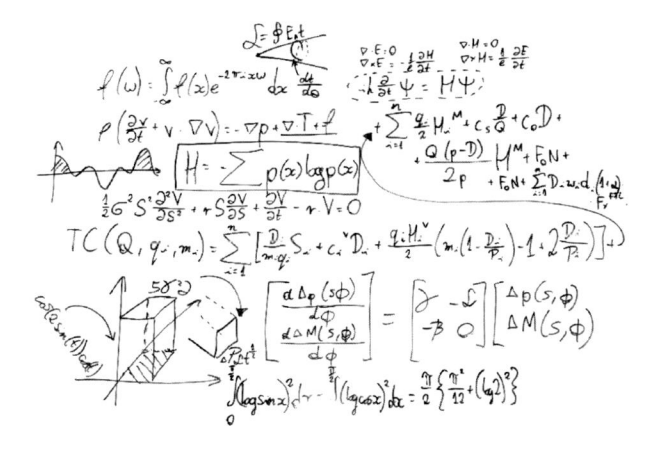

Calorie counting is more about calorie estimating or guessing.

Even though it's possible to quantify the calories in a packaged food, and you can estimate the calorie expenditure of a workout, it's important to keep in mind that calorie tracking is always a bit of a mystery. You'll never be able to track either calorie intake or expenditure very accurately without substantial cost. The good news is you don't have to be an expert calorie counter.

Remember, it's the balance between intake and expenditure that's in charge. It doesn't matter what the numbers are. The most important thing is the ratio between those readings.

"Eat less and move more" does not mean "eat right and exercise"

The talk about calorie balance inevitably brings up the age old recommendation of "eat less and move more." Even though it's an old rule, it's usually pretty sound advice. If you start off with a calorie balance and decrease your caloric intake while increasing your caloric expenditure, you stand an excellent chance of tipping that calorie balance to cause fat loss. Even though it's a simple piece of advice eat less and move more is often criticized for being too simple or an old outdated way of thinking. Some even claim it simply doesn't work.

Possibly the biggest issue is "eat less and move more" often gets misinterpreted as "eat right and exercise." Even though the two phrases sound similar, they mean very different things. Whereas eating less and moving more is about tipping the calorie balance, eating right and exercising may or may not cause a shift in calorie balance because it's focusing on satisfying a few limited influences as opposed to the cause.

I go into more detail about the issue of "eating right" later on, but the general idea is that eating right is about adhering to a dietary rule such as eating the right kinds of foods or staying away from other certain foods. Meanwhile, exercising often means being active in a gym or attending some fitness class. It doesn't always mean you're significantly increasing your calorie expenditure.

Let's use abstaining from bread and attending a weekly fitness class as an example. While cutting out bread and doing a class can influence your calorie balance, it's possible to stick to those habits and not cause a fat shedding negative calorie balance. Maybe you've replaced the bread calories with something else like rice or meat. Exercising is an excellent way to increase your T.E.A, but since it's only influence, it's still possible to keep the same level of calorie expenditure throughout the week by being a little less active outside of your workouts.

So while "eat less and move more" means to decrease intake and increase expenditure, sticking to a few dietary rules and getting in a workout are no guarantee that will happen. Thus, when "eat less and move more" gets turned into "eat right and exercise" the emphasis shifts away from altering your calorie balance to fulfilling a few select influences which leave your control over the cause in doubt.

I too didn't believe in calorie balance

I don't blame anyone for being skeptical about calorie balance. After all, I was a skeptic for many years myself. I always thought fat levels boiled down to insulin control or metabolism boosting workout programs. The thing that ultimately changed my mind was when I realized that every fat loss theory came down to a calorie balance.... even when that very theory claimed it wasn't.

When I started to take a hard look at trending fat loss methods, I adopted the same approach a curious little kid might take. I would ask why that diet or workout plan would work and then I asked "why" after every answer I got. Why did increase in metabolism matter? Why did eating foods that took more work to break down matter? After a few years of searching, I figured that almost all fat loss methods work because you either eat less or expending more calories. Despite all of the latest research, every diet or workout strategy was just another roundabout way of getting you to decrease your calorie intake or increase your calorie expenditure.

The only trouble is that fat loss depends on the *balance* between calories in and calories out and most methods only deal with one side of that balance. Even if a single diet or workout program can be a significant influence, it can still fall short of controlling the balance because your intake or expenditure is only one-half of the cause. In an attempt to make up for this shortcoming, the most efficient methods are typically those that have the most influence on their half of that balance. So the plans that dealt with calorie expenditure had to ensure you burned a lot of calories to increase the chances of success. The plans that dealt with calorie intake had to reduce significantly the amount of food you could eat, so the influence was significant enough to produce results.

While a bigger influence does increase your chance of tipping your energy balance, it also increases the demand for your lifestyle resources. The result is trying to control your fat levels through just caloric expenditure or intake can become a very costly, and stressful. When you manipulate a few influences on both sides of the balance, you gain far more control over the entire cause giving you the power to achieve better results through less cost.

Yes! You can out train a bad diet. You probably already do

It's very popular for trainers and fat loss coaches to claim you can't out-train a bad diet. In other words, no matter how much you exercise you'll never get anywhere if your diet sucks. The statement is an attempt to pull some focus away from calorie expenditure and placing more emphasis on the intake half of the calorie balance. The problem is it holds the risk of over-emphasizing calorie intake and trivializing calorie expenditure. The idea you can't out train a bad diet has swung the pendulum so far to the food half of the calorie balance that some people even claim diet is the lion's share of fat loss. This idea is nothing more than delusional thinking. Diet is never 80 or 90% of your success in fat loss. Diet is only responsible for your calorie intake which is responsible for only 50% of your calorie balance and thus any changes in weight.

The only reason why a change in diet can result in the fat loss is how that change influences your calorie intake in relation to your calorie output. If you change your diet and lose weight it's not because of your diet; it's because how that diet influenced your calorie intake while the effect of calorie expenditure kept your fat burning furnace fired up. So yes, you certainly can "out train a bad diet." Chances are you already do it every day. On the other hand, it's impossible to out train a bad diet out no matter what you do. Let me explain.

First, let's be honest about what "a bad diet" really means. A bad diet doesn't cause weight gain. A truly bad diet causes malnutrition when people can't eat enough to sustain a healthy body. Chances are if you're trying to get six pack abs or lose 20 pounds you don't need to worry too much about an actual bad diet. After all, you don't hear of many cases of scurvy or rickets among people who can afford gym memberships and vitamin pills. In the event of such malnutrition, no, you can't out-train a bad diet. If someone is suffering from a vitamin deficiency, they will continue to suffer no matter how much they run or how many pushups they do.

When someone claims you can't out train, a bad diet chances are they are not talking about malnutrition. They are not thinking about a bad diet but rather a *fattening* diet which is a very different case. A fattening diet is one that involves a calorie intake that promotes weight gain or prevents fat loss. A fattening diet happens when your calorie intake is high in relation to your calorie expenditure. The problem is, the term "bad diet" is used to convey the idea that the excess calorie intake is due to the influences of certain foods people claim are fattening. Sometimes when someone cuts those foods out of their diet, the impact causes a drop in calorie intake and thus influencing the calorie balance to cause fat loss.

There's nothing wrong with changing your diet in an attempt to initiate fat loss. It's a very smart thing to do when you're in the first few weeks of a fat loss plan. The issue I want to address is making the mistake in believing your activity level can't have a substantial influence towards your fat loss while acknowledging that while diet is important, it's not *that* potent for fat loss.

Of course, you can out train a fattening diet. If you are physically active, yet are not losing weight, that means you're maintaining a calorie balance because of the calories you're burning through your physical activity. If you were to suddenly stop expending those calories, yet maintain your current diet you would gain weight.

This sort of thing happens quite often when someone who is very active suddenly finds themselves much less active due to injury or a change in lifestyle. A typical example is when a college athlete stops practicing their sport when they start working. If they maintain the diet they had in school, they will likely find themselves gaining body fat because their activity level is no longer holding them in calorie balance. The result is, their old diet was indeed a potentially fattening diet, but it only became fattening when they became more sedentary and was no longer out training their potentially fattening diet.

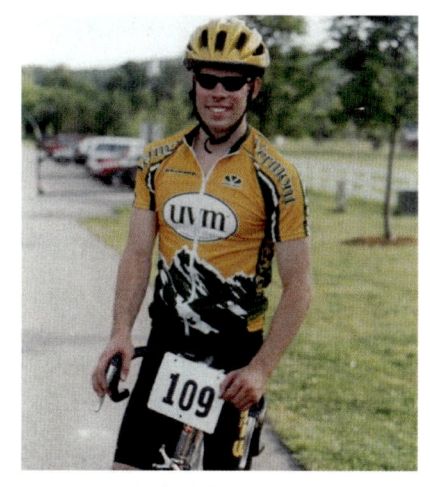

I out-trained a bad diet every day while racing bikes in college.

The idea that you can't out train a bad diet is best used to illustrate the idea that it's a lot easier to cut calories out of your diet than it is to work them off. In essence, you can spend 2 hours trying to run off a big bowl of ice cream, or you can simply not eat the ice cream in the first place. However, if you're trying to lose weight you certainly do want to increase your calorie expenditure as much as possible. After all, your body can only burn so much energy on a given day no matter how you eat. Relying mostly on a diet to lose weight is a limited approach. While it can work, why try to control body fat through only one-half of the calorie balance when you can potentially influence both halves and make progress a lot easier, not to mention more effective?

Besides, it is most certainly possible to lose body fat primarily through exercise. I've done it, and I've known other people who've done it. The only problem is it takes a lot more work than many individuals are willing to invest. Back when I was training for the U.V.M cycling team, I was eating more in a single day than most people would eat in two or even three days. On top of that, much of my food was highly processed and loaded with simple sugars, yet I was always very lean. My secret was simple; I was riding my bike as hard as I could 1-2 hours every day, taking 20,000 steps around campus and racing 4-6 hours every weekend. I was so active I hardly even sat down to study. I was always reading a book or looking at my notes as I pedaled away on an exercise bike.

According to modern fat loss theories, my diet back then should have been as fattening as ever, but it wasn't because I was "out training it" every day. Was it easy? Hell no! Sometimes it even made me fight bouts of exhaustion, but the point is it worked.

The real calorie balance myth

The funny thing about a negative calorie imbalance is that it's impossible to create. No matter what, your body is always expending the same number of calories it consumes. When I mentioned that you consume calories from food and drink I left out one other source of calories - your body. Your body has fat, protein and carbohydrate just like any foodstuff you may eat. Of course, you get all of those calorie sources from food in the first place. However, when I talk about a negative calorie balance, I'm referring to fewer calories coming from food and more coming from your body.

For example, if you burn 2,500 calories per day you absolutely must consume 2,500 calories each day. There is no caloric line of credit your body can take out so that it can burn calories it doesn't have available. The amount of caloric energy you consume and spend is always the same. The only difference is the source of the calories you're burning. This basic idea points out a simple, yet striking fact about calorie balance and body weight. If you burn more calories than you consume from food, then you *must* make up the difference from your stored calories. When this happens, your body weight will drop without exception.

Sometimes, experts will tell people that something is wrong when they believe they burn 2,500 calories a day but they only eat 1,500 a day, yet they don't lose weight. If they are not in a calorie balance why are they not losing weight?

Some experts will point to burning muscle or a slowing metabolism. While there is some science to suggest this is the cause of the discrepancy, it's missing the bigger yet more evident fact. If the person's body weight is the same, their caloric balance has returned. It's physiologically impossible to burn more calories than you eat or drink and not lose weight. You must make up that difference from your body and when you do you will lose weight.

Sometimes people will claim the person is not burning fat but rather muscle tissue. As scary as that may seem, even that should result in weight loss. If anything, it should lead to losing, even *more,* weight. If fat has roughly nine calories per gram and protein has only four calories per gram that means there's over twice as much weight per unit of energy with protein compared to fat. So if you're burning muscle to make up that calorie balance, you should be losing at least twice as much weight! Carbohydrate also has about four calories per gram. You may lose even more body weight since carbohydrate is also known to hold onto water, maybe as much as 3-4 grams of it.

The bottom line is that if you're not eating as much as your body is expending, then you must make up the difference from the energy stored in your body and that's Impossible to do without a drop in body weight. While our efforts to account for every calorie may be highly fallible, our body is always dead on accurate. Even if your calorie charts and electronic devices say you're in a negative calorie balance, the actual condition of your body is always a valid and accurate way to monitor your calorie balance.

I also fully acknowledge that there's always a lot more to the story than calorie readouts. Solving the calorie mystery requires a lot more than adjusting how much you eat or move around during the day. Sometimes there are emotional reasons behind eating a lot, which I'll get a little more into later on. Other times there could be a medical issue or hormonal change going on that is influencing the balance. My goal in writing this chapter isn't to make weight management seem straightforward and easy because it's often not. Instead, understanding the root is simply the foundation to base your further research all the while preventing you from getting distracted by influential over-reliance.

5: The Cause of Training Muscle

Next to fat, muscle is one of the most sought after goals in our fitness culture. Growing stronger is a good thing, especially considering the health and condition of your muscles can have a vast influence over your overall fitness. I would even argue that when it comes to your health and performance muscle is far more important when compared to body fat. The condition of your muscle tissue is holding the keys to helping you look, feel and perform your best for the following reasons.

1. **Muscle helps your body look great**

Unless you have a lot of body fat to burn off, improving the condition of your muscles will do far more to improve your appearance than fat loss ever will. If you lose some body fat, your body will only be a smaller version of what you looked like before. While that will help you fit into your skinny jeans, it's muscle tissue that gives your body most of its shape and curves.

While the shape of your physique is important in helping you look your best, it pales in comparison to the importance of how you use your muscles to present your physique. It doesn't matter how lean you look, or how big your muscles are; how you *use* your body speaks volumes to anyone who looks your way.

Your shoulders and back strength might tell the world you're strong and confident or easily intimidated. How you walk or use your arms can shout to everyone around that you're strong and powerful or weak and frail. It's all influenced by the subtle ways you present your body through the strength you develop in your muscles. You don't have to be a big bodybuilder to look strong and confident, nor do you have to be skinny like a model to appear beautiful and sexy. In fact, you could have the muscles or the beautiful face, but your body language can still overshadow those influences.

Even more important, the way you carry yourself is often an unconscious habit you can't just decide to turn on or off. It's a reflection of how you use your body every single day. This powerful presence is not something you can quickly adopt or fake. While big biceps may draw attention, your posture has a powerful, yet the subliminal effect on everyone you meet. It's almost like a Jedi mind trick when you have a strong back or powerful legs. People won't know exactly why you're healthy and attractive they'll just know it when they see it.

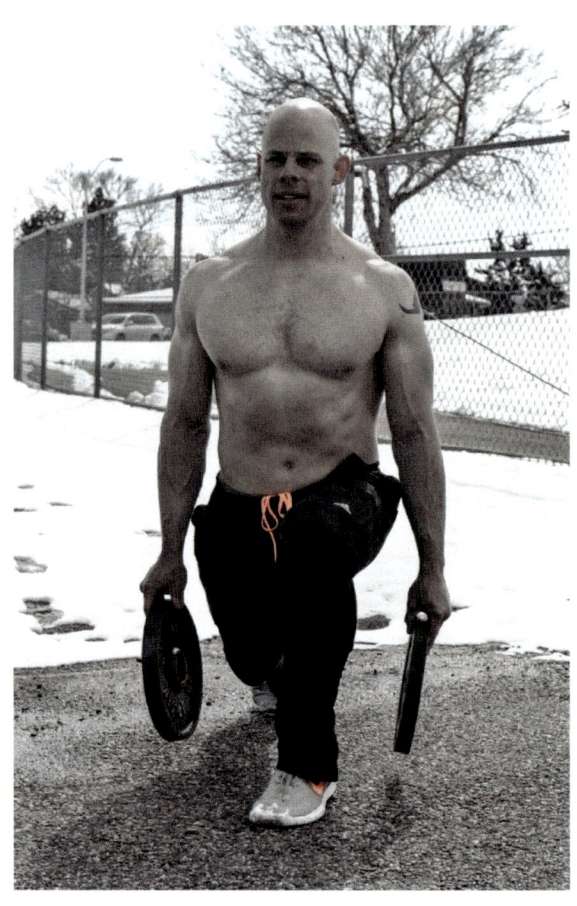

Just having muscle isn't enough. It's how you use your muscle that's most important.

Lastly, muscle helps you look your best through helping you burn fat. Simply put, fully capable muscles make it easier to burn a lot of fat and calories. If your muscles are not well conditioned, all physical activity will require much more effort on your part to expend the same amount of energy as someone with much stronger muscles. Just consider someone who's weak and has trouble moving around. Even climbing a single flight of stairs can be a daunting task prompting them to take the elevator. In contrast, someone who's stronger can run up three flights of stairs and hardly be out of breath. That person will have a much easier time increasing their calorie expenditure making it easier to lose and maintain their body fat levels.

2. **Muscle keeps you young and healthy**

Muscle is the real fountain of youth. Almost every affliction threatening you in old age can be traced directly to the condition of your muscles. Everything from being able to move around to avoiding falls comes down to how strong you are.

Its more than just being able to climb stairs and avoiding a bone-breaking fall. The health of your muscular system heavily influences many other systems in your body. Everything from your bone strength, the health of your joints and even the condition of your blood is affected by your muscular conditioning.

You can see evidence in the link between muscle and health in any physical therapy clinic. Just walk in and you'll find people suffering from a wide range of issues from injury and illness to recovery from surgery. In almost all cases you'll find people doing exercises designed to challenge their ability to use their muscles. The physical therapists understand that when the muscles become better trained, the problem will cease to exist. It's proof that using your muscle is the best medicine out there.

3. **Muscle is the primary key to your performance**

Your muscle is much more important towards your performance than your body fat level. There isn't a single physical activity you can succeed at with weak and poorly developed muscles. Losing a few pounds of fat might, or might not, improve your performance, but becoming active will always pay high dividends on the field, the court or the trail.

I've just scratched the surface, but I think I've made my point. Muscle is a pretty big deal concerning your fitness, health, performance and overall quality of life. Even though fat loss is a major market within our fitness culture, muscle is more important towards your health and fitness.

The high cost of muscle

In light of the vast importance of being strong, it's a wonder why many people don't focus on conditioning their muscles. One reason could be the antiquated idea that cardio is the most important training for fat loss. Another reason could be the equally old idea that strength training means building large and over developed muscles, something only a few people may want. Like many hurdles in fitness, I believe the biggest challenge facing muscle training boils down to cost. Modern muscle conditioning is often extremely costly. It requires a lot of time, money, and other lifestyle resources for various reasons.

The first reason is the vast selection of possible exercises you can do to "attack" every muscle in your body. You can move your body in an infinite number of ways setting up the potential to make a massive selection of exercises. Each exercise requires your time and energy. All of those exercises have also spawned countless equipment choices ranging from different machines to a plethora of free weight options. Having access to the "necessary" equipment means you have to buy the equipment yourself, or spend money every month for a gym membership. In either case, you're talking about spending a lot of money for a lot of various toys that you now have to spend a lot of time and energy to use.

It's not just the exercises and equipment that cost you a lot, but building muscle is often coupled with costly diet practices as well. This includes supplements ranging from amino acid pills and protein powder to pre-workout shakes. When I was younger, I thought I was a serious athlete because I drank a protein shake after a workout. These days there's stuff to take before your workout, during your workout, after your workout and any other time of day.

Outside of supplements, food preparation is also a costly part of building muscle. Some people plan and prepare as many as 6 or 7 meals a day in the mistaken belief they need to eat very frequently or else their body will start breaking down their muscle with blinding speed.
Due to these high costs, it's easy to see why, even though, conditioning your muscles yields many rewards, it can become very costly pretty darn quick plus I haven't even told you the worst part yet!

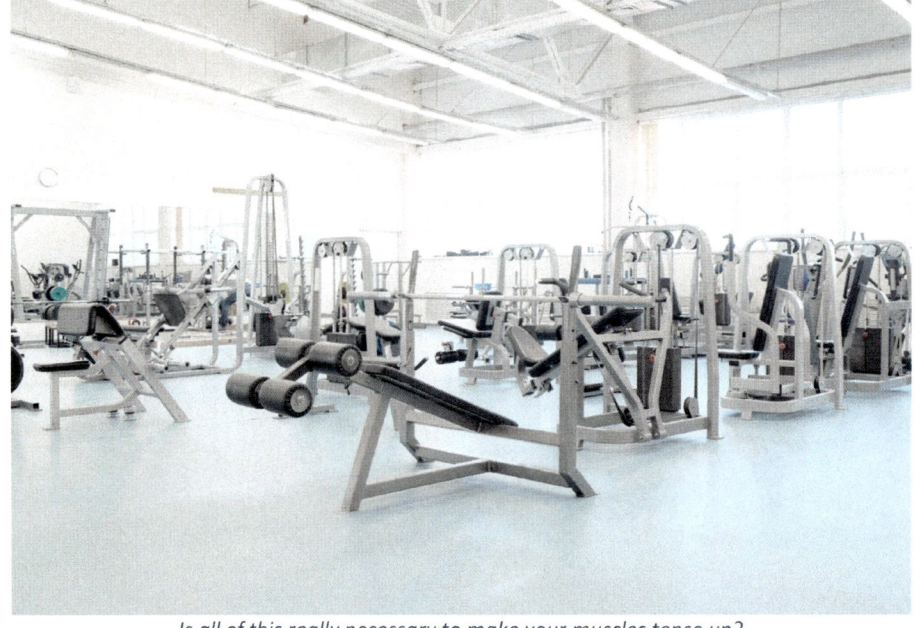

Is all of this really necessary to make your muscles tense up?

Maintaining a healthy body is not like keeping a lean body. You can work hard to lose fat, but once you are lean all you need to do is maintain your calorie balance, and you never have to worry about becoming overweight ever again. Unfortunately, conditioning muscle is not like this. To build, and then maintain your muscle you have to continue your habits indefinitely.

When you stop doing your exercises, your body automatically assumes you no longer need that power, and your gains melt away. So not only is muscle expensive to build but it's a never ending expense you are required to continue paying. It doesn't matter if your life changes or you can no longer afford the costly methods. You must keep paying the high price or else you will lose all of your progress very quickly.

It kind of sounds like a no-win scenario doesn't it? It's no wonder many people become stronger and more capable for a short period and then stop and lose their results. Many people won't bother starting at all. Many are satisfied with just losing weight and calling it a day there. After all, they may be mistakenly struggling just to lose the weight and keep it off, why add a whole new costly project to the mix?

Muscle doesn't have to cost you so much time and energy!

You don't have to spend an arm and a leg to train your muscle. You probably don't even need 90% of the costs commonly associated with exercising for muscle in the first place. Just as with all aspects of Fitness Independence, the key to gaining far more from far less is understanding the cause of all things muscle.

The cause of muscle

Muscle is a functional tissue. It's responsible for most of the bodily functions you consciously control. Since it's a functional tissue, muscle responds to the demands you place upon it. It doesn't change or adapt for any odd reason. It's just like the skin on your hands. You're not going to build calluses just because you take a supplement or eat a particular type of protein. Your skin only adapts because of the functional demand placed upon it. If you start doing manual labor that stresses the skin on your hands, your hands will change according to that demand and thicken the skin. Your muscles develop for the same reason. Supply the demand and your muscles will follow suit. However, you can spend all of the resources in the world but if the functional demand isn't there your muscles will never change.

The logical question then is what creates the signals telling the muscles what to do? I used to believe the request on my muscles came from a heavy weight or a supplement, but I couldn't have been more wrong. The demand on your muscles doesn't originate from a source external to your body. It comes from your mind.

The mind-muscle signal

I once met a weightlifter who had a bicep that looked like a deflated balloon. This guy was doing curls like a madman yet no matter how hard he worked his left bicep still looked flat. We got to talking, and it turned out he had suffered some nerve damage in his shoulder which prevented one of his biceps muscles from fully activating. He asked me if there was anything he could do for it and over the next hour we tried every bicep exercise in the gym. Nothing worked even a little. I went home and did some research. The next day I met him and delivered the somber news; unless he could repair the nerve in his shoulder, there was absolutely nothing he could do. No gadget, technique or supplement could bring his bicep back.

It was through this little event that I began to explore the cause with all things muscle. What we're dealing with isn't just the muscle tissue itself but the physical system that's responsible for making the muscle operate. As my weight lifting friend learned, if something interferes with that system the necessary demand on the muscle will not happen. Let's explore this system by starting at the muscle and working backward.

Your neuromuscular system

Your muscles are made up of muscle fibers which have two settings; off and on. A muscle fiber can't halfway contract; it's either fully contracted or fully relaxed. It's just like those computers I was checking out at the history museum in Silicon Valley. Computers run on a binary system of 1s and 0s. Your muscles operate the same way.

The 2 Stages of a Muscle Fiber

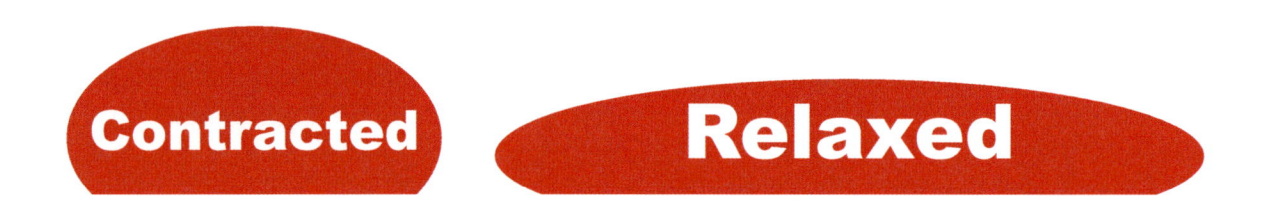

Contracted **Relaxed**

Moving up the system, your binary muscle fibers "plug into" a neuron. I like to think of a neuron-like a light socket and the muscle fibers plug into it like light bulbs. Some neurons have a few muscle fibers, and these are responsible for smaller movements like the movement in your eye. Other neurons have many muscle fibers like the strong movements of your legs. In either case, all of the muscle fibers on that single neuron either all turn on or off. The muscle fibers and their associated neuron are collectively known as a motor unit.

Since your muscles operate on a binary system, everything you do from shaking your head to throwing a javelin comes from a particular signal running through your nervous system telling certain motor units to contract their muscle fibers in a very specific sequence. It's this coded signal that created the demand upon your muscle tissue.

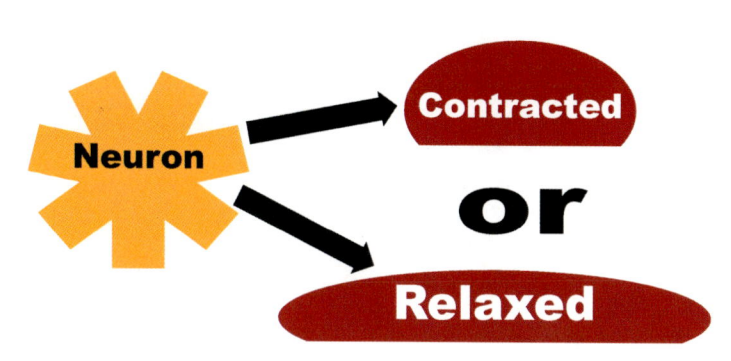

Motor Unit

All physical movement depends upon which motor units you use to engage their associated muscle fibers.

Logically, the next important question is what creates the all-important muscle programming signal? Just as you can find the source of a river by moving upstream, you can locate the origin of the muscle controlling signal by moving up your nervous system. From the neurons in your muscles, you travel through your peripheral nervous system which runs to your spinal cord. Finally, you move up your spine to the source of all muscle signals which is your brain.

So working back down, the signal originates in your brain, travels down your spinal cord, branches out through your peripheral nervous system; hits a particular set of neurons and the muscle fibers associated with those neurons contract to create the functional demand you want.

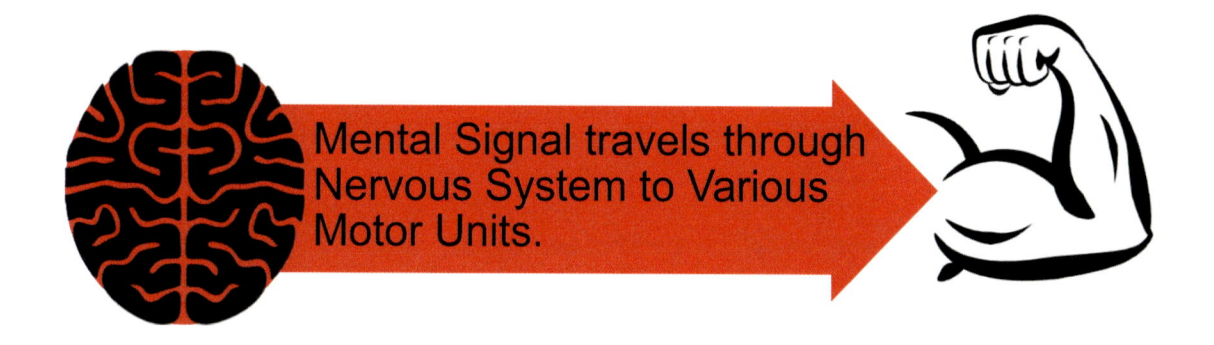

Mental Signal travels through Nervous System to Various Motor Units.

The mental signal starts in your brain where it travels down your spinal cord and is distributed throughout your nervous system to various neurons which make their associated muscle fibers contract.

The cool thing is the mind-muscle connection is a 2-way street. Not only does your mind send signals to your muscles, but it can also receive feedback based on what your muscles are doing. This feedback is critical for helping you refine that mind-muscle signal so it can become more efficient at producing the result you want.

This cycle of instructions and feedback is the essence of what makes your muscles do what they do. It's the cause responsible for everything from driving a golf ball off the tee to telling your muscles to become stronger. Everything you want to accomplish resides within that signal telling your muscles what they should do and the feedback they are sending back.

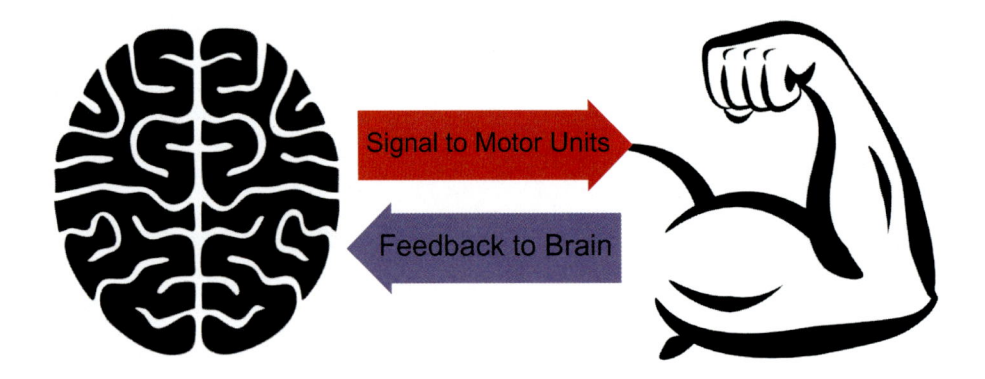

The practice of training is nothing more than refining the signal that cycles between your mind and your muscles.

You can sense this cycle in action if you've ever tried to become proficient in an activity like shooting a basketball or riding a bike. On your first few attempts, your mind is trying to make your body do something. With each attempt, your mind receives feedback based on how well you did. From there, your mind will slightly adjust the signal, so you change use your muscles a little differently and do better the next time around. After many repetitions, the message has become refined to the point where your muscles are performing the task you want to with a high degree of proficiency.

Lessons from the cause of muscle conditioning

The mind-muscle connection might seem simple enough, but it brings some fascinating facts to light about your training and the purpose behind your exercise.

1. **It's not about the tools you use, but how your muscles use them**

When you look at the cause of muscle, you'll notice that something is missing. There's nothing in there about supplements, equipment, workouts, or any of these other things that are supposedly so darn important. All of the weights, tools, and products you buy are nothing more than influences that help you create the appropriate signal in your mind. If a product affects how your brain uses your muscle, then it has some value. However, if a product doesn't make your mind improve how it's engaging your muscles, it's pretty close to worthless. Nothing you buy can make your muscles do anything. Only your mind can do that thus anything that's going to help you train your muscles must influence your mind.

2. **Training isn't just working out**

The terms training and working out may mean the same thing to most people, but to me; they couldn't be more different. Training is the purposeful practice of trying to refine the mental instructions coming from the mind so the muscles are used in a better way. Just think back to when you were learning to ride a bike. Your mind was concentrating on staying upright on your bike. Every minute of your practice was involved in making the instructions coming from your mind a little more tuned in to help you accomplish your goals.

In comparison, working out usually lacks such a high level of mental focus. It's when you're making your body work hard for the sake of using your body under stress. Maybe you're running on a treadmill to burn calories or going through the motions in a workout routine someone planned out for you. In either case, your mind is just getting the job done as opposed to looking for ways to do it better.

While working out can produce some results, the act of training to improve your muscle controlling mental signal is where your success truly exists. Working out will produce some results, but you'll only go as far as your mental know-how will allow. If you keep exercising the same way, the mental signal will never change, and your progress will stall no matter how hard you work. When you consciously train, your mind will always be learning how to do the exercise better, and your muscles continue to receive new instructions how they should behave. As long as you keep learning, you'll never truly plateau in your workouts.

3. Training is trying

The Star Wars character, Yoda, is famous for saying "Do or do not, there is no try." It's funny because everything he had Luke Skywalker doing in the movie is about try, try and try again. The very act of trying to do something is what causes your mind-muscle signal to become refined and more efficient towards making your muscles do what you want. This is why every effective workout is all about trying to improve what you're doing. Maybe you're trying to do one more rep, or you're trying to run a little smoother. As long as you're trying to do something a little better your muscles will continue to adapt.

4. Distractions prevent you from training

Distraction is the poison that interferes with your training. When your mind is thinking about replying to a Facebook feed or the latest news story your ability to concentrate on improving that mental signal is substantially diminished. The funny thing is, distractions are very popular in fitness these days. People love to watch TV or gossip when exercising as a way to pass the time.

What they don't know is these distractions are interfering with the very purpose of their training.
You don't have to eliminate all distractions when training. That can be impractical if not impossible in some circumstances. The key is to reduce distractions as much as possible so you can continuously concentrate on what you're doing.

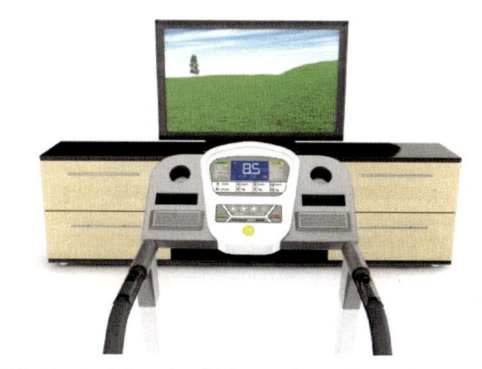

Effective training shouldn't require a distraction.

5. Modifying your mental signal kills boredom

Boredom is one of the biggest challenges fitness enthusiasts face. This boredom is one of the biggest reasons people seek distractions to keep their mind occupied. When your mind is focusing on continually improving the way you use your muscles boredom is squelched. After all, you can't be bored if you're trying very hard to keep your heels down as you squat or when trying for a personal best of how many pushups you can do in a minute.

6. Skill based exercise is best

The past few decades have seen the growth of many technologies that have attempted to remove the skill factor from exercise. Simple weight machines and cardio equipment make working out easy for almost anyone. The issue with these simple forms of training is twofold. First, equipment that requires less skill to use is often more expensive to use. You either need to purchase the gear yourself or belong to a gym and shackle yourself to a monthly membership fee, not to mention the cost of getting to and from the gym.

The second issue is since these methods don't require a lot of skill to use, your mind quickly becomes accustomed to the exercise. Without anything new to challenge you, boredom can quickly set in. Since the mind doesn't refine the instructions it is sending to the muscles, both body and mind fall into a routine that lacks any stimulation for change. The same signals are sent to the muscles over and over and although this helps maintain current levels of conditioning; it makes progress almost impossible.

I'm a big fan of skill based exercise methods because they inherently encourage you to keep improving your mental signal. The tools and exercises that require the most skill also happen to come at the lowest cost. Advanced bodyweight training is a great example. You don't need a gym and hardly any equipment, yet you can spend years trying to master moves like the one arm push up and hill sprints.

The S.A.I.D principle

The S.A.I.D principle just may be the single most important rule in all of fitness and exercise science. Once you understand the S.A.I.D principle, you'll know about 90% of everything you'll ever need to know about how to train towards any objective. To see why the S.A.I.D principle is so important to let's go back to the anatomy lesson where I mentioned your muscle fibers are attached to a neuron and together they are known as a Motor Unit.

Everything you do, from typing on a keyboard to pushing a car out of a ditch is all about what motor units your mind is firing off and in what sequence. I like to think of using motor units sort of like keys on a piano keyboard. Playing a piece of music requires you to strike certain keys in a certain order with precise timing. If you hit the right keys, at the right time, then you get a very specific piece of music. If you want a different piece of music, you need to hit those keys in a different order with different timing.

Moving your body is just like playing that piano where your motor units are the keys, only now you have millions of keys instead of just 88. The use of your motor units is very specific to the activity you do. If you change even the slightest aspect of the exercise you shift what motor units are working and the order in which they are contracting their muscle fibers. It's all very specific to what you're doing which is why they call it the *Specific* Adaptation to Imposed Demand or the S.A.I.D principle.

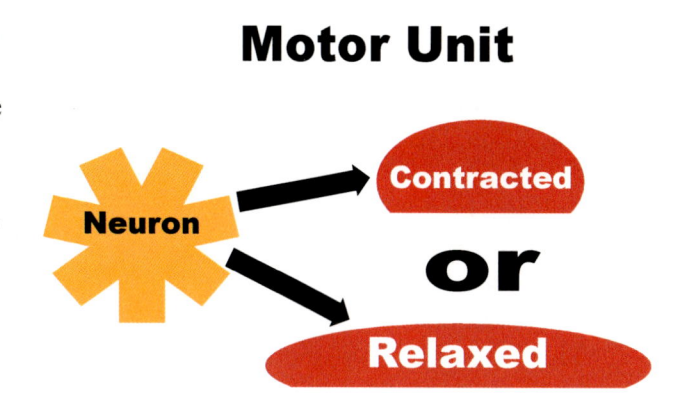

Everything you do fires your motor units in a very specific way thus the adaptations your body go through are also specific to that activity. Every exercise you do is your mind telling your body "HEY! Be able to do this thing exactly this way." It's a simple principle but there are some profound lessons to learn about fitness and exercise.

S.A.I.D Lesson #1 All training is about function

People exercise for various reasons, and some of those reasons are to improve the appearance of the body. There's nothing wrong with working out to burn off some calories or build some muscle but the S.A.I.D principle teaches us that such objectives are just side effects to the real purpose of any and all exercise which is functional capability.

The Specific Adaptation to Imposed Demand doesn't happen so you can be leaner or have bigger arms. The adaptations your body goes through are due to the particular *functional* demand of the exercise or activity and nothing more. In other words, function and capability are the only reason why your body changes in any and all forms of training.

The functional demand of activity explains why there is no such thing as a fat loss or "toning" exercise. The signal coming from your mind has only one objective, and that's to get your body to *do* something. Function is the one and only thing your body understands. When you're on the elliptical, you may be training for endurance or a marathon, but the only signal your body receives is that it needs to become proficient at using an elliptical. If you're on a bicep curl weight machine, you're training your body to be proficient at using a bicep curl machine. You might have other motivations for doing those exercises, but as far as Mother Nature knows, you're just training your body to be able to do that activity.

Also, remember you're not only training to do those exercises, but you're also training to do those exercises that particular way. So if you're using a Precor elliptical for 20 minutes on level 8, then you're conditioning yourself to use a Precor elliptical for 20 minutes on level 8. If you change your position on the machine that will slightly change the particular demand of the exercise.

S.A.I.D Lesson #2 Functional carry over

Functional carryover is when you do an exercise that has a functional demand that's similar to an activity you're looking to excel in. The key is in understanding what those demands are and matching them up with your activity.

A classic example is in my Taekwondo sparring class. Inevitably, at least one new student will become winded and tired after a few rounds of sparring. They don't understand how they can run for miles, yet become exhausted after 2 minutes of sparring.

While running and sparring will both make you out of breath, they have limited functional carryover from one to the other. Running seven miles requires a sustained effort for more than 30 minutes and the movement is short and repetitive. Sparring, on the other hand, lasts only a short time, includes many quick bursts of all-out effort and requires a variety of techniques. So while running and sparring will crank up your heart rate, it's clear to see how long distance running would fall short of sparring and sparring would fall short of long distance running. There isn't a lot of functional carryover between the two activities. On the other hand, if you were to prepare for a 5K charity race, seven miles of running would be a great way to prepare yourself.

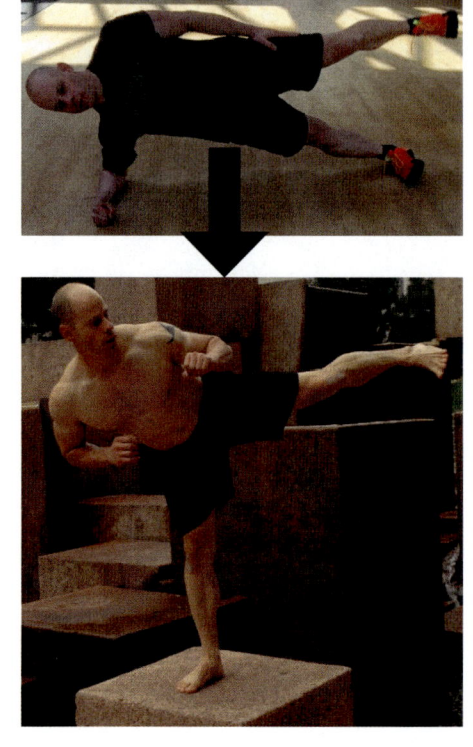

As far as the sparring might be concerned, an exercise with a lot of carryover to sparring might be to punch and kick a heavy bag in timed rounds. It's not exactly sparring, but the physical demands on the body would be similar to sparring and thus have far more functional carryover.

Always look for the functional carry-over from an exercise to the activity you want to improve.

Functional carryover also applies in any form of strength training. A bench press might not be the most functional way to condition you for hiking up a mountain. However, if you have a bench press competition coming up then it's very useful and practical. The real question isn't so much about what exercises are functional or nonfunctional, but rather what exercises have the most functional carryover for what you want to do.

S.A.I.D Lesson #3 You gain what you challenge

The S.A.I.D principle makes it simple to figure out how to train towards any goal. As I mentioned before, you can prepare your body by getting your mind to try to do something. To put it another way, you gain whatever you challenge when it comes to functional ability. So if you want to improve your speed do exercises that challenge your speed. If you want to train for more endurance, challenge your stamina. If you want more grip strength, then test your ability to grasp onto something. If you challenge it, your mind will send a stronger signal to your body on how it should behave and your body will adapt accordingly every time.

Once again, notice that this applies to the capabilities of the body. You can't challenge being skinny or toned nor can you challenge a V-shaped torso or longer legs. You can only directly challenge functional capability.

S.A.I.D Lesson #4 Set functional priorities

The S.A.I.D principle forces you to be efficient with your training and the use of your lifestyle resources. Training is a costly endeavor and requires some of your finite resources. So while you can train yourself very well towards any function, you can't optimally train for everything. The need to prioritize training is why you don't see athletes who are the world's best cyclist, power lifter, bowler and high jumper. Each of these activities requires lifestyle resources, and the more you spend towards one goal, the less you have to devote to the others. You can become proficient at doing anything; you just can't become great at doing everything.

Being limited in your goals isn't a bad thing. It means you have permission to pursue the activities you enjoy doing and are important to you. In my case, I'm an avid mountain biker and skier. I love doing those things, and I'm reasonably proficient at them. On the other hand, I can't run worth a damn. If I run a 5K, I won't be able to walk for a week. I'm in terrible shape for running, and I know it, but, that's okay.

Thanks to our modern society, I don't have to be a good runner. If I don't want to spend the resources to become a good runner, then I don't have to. Beware that our fitness culture doesn't like to tell you that it's okay to be out of shape for something. Many will claim you're not in shape if you can't adhere to their own performance standards. I've had people tell me that I'm not fit because I don't run or swim very well. I've had some folks claim that I'm not strong because I don't bench press or practice Olympic lifting. I could make the same argument though about their ability to do one leg squats or how fast they can hike up the local mountain.

There is no standard of performance when it comes to fitness as a whole. We are all weak and out of shape in some areas and strong in others. Some people like to look down on others as a way to feel better. Like all forms of criticism, this comes from personal insecurity. It's nothing about you; it's all about them. Feel free to pick and choose the standards that apply to your requirements and preferences. As long as you know what you want and are getting it then, that's all that matters.

S.A.I.D Lesson #5 Only you can be in charge

Ultimately, the cause of muscle teaches that all muscle tension can only come from your mind. As a personal trainer, I can't make anyone run faster or jump higher. The most I can do is tell them what to work on. The person I'm working with must create the signals in their mind and send those messages to their muscles. I can't make it happen for them.

So that's the long and the short of training your muscles. It doesn't matter if you're trying to improve your golf swing or improve your posture, everything boils down to what your mind is telling your muscles. The better you refine that mental signal, the better your results will be guaranteed. Through challenging the functional characteristics you want, you're sure to become more fit and capable towards any goal.

6: The Cause of Bodybuilding / Shaping

Interest in sculpting the human body has reached an almost obsessive level within our fitness culture. You can hardly turn on a TV or glimpse a newsstand without being blasted by programs that promise to shape, sculpt, mold and carve your body as if it were made of clay.

I find this obsession with using diet and exercise to improve the shape of the body fascinating because it's a very modern idea. Even though the marketing behind such an idea is prolific, the human body didn't evolve to change its appearance in reliable ways from working out and eating right. Yes, you read that correctly. I'm claiming the idea that fitness can be a credible body shaping vehicle is more a product of our imagination than truthful fact. Mother Nature never intended the physical adaptations from diet and exercise to be directly responsible for a change in appearance.

The birth of the fitness = appearance myth

The widespread use of fitness as a means to sculpt the body is a very new concept that's grown from hype and inflated promises. To understand how all of these promises came about let's examine a brief history of how humans have related to physical adaptation over time.

Fitness and physical change is the result of a long evolutionary journey that predates any diet or exercise methods in use today. Getting in shape has never been about working out in a gym or looking good for a wedding. Instead, fitness has always been about function and utility which is something far more fundamental towards survival. Before our modern fitness culture, people didn't work their muscles to get pumped up or to score points in a game. Everything from hunting to fighting to travel and even entertainment used the body as a tool to accomplish a task. Every inch of your physique from the bones in your shoulder to the way your muscles work has evolved for the single purpose to be able to do stuff.

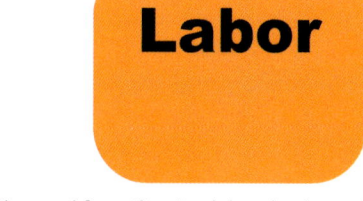

The need for utilitarian labor dominated all physical activity for most of human history.

The birth of civilization caused people to start using their body in progressive ways. Over time, some workers began to specialize in skill-based labor like performance arts and fighting. As these specialized professions developed, It was no longer enough to just be a hunter, now people trained to be a *better* hunter. The need to become progressively better spawned the first exercise revolution.

People learned how to condition their body so they could perform at a higher level through systematic training. They had become a subculture within society known as the athlete. As civilization continued to develop, the athletic subculture continued to progress and learned to develop extraordinary levels of performance. People learned how to condition the body through manipulating various influences to control their physical capability. This stage lasted through most of recorded human history.

The next great social change came from the industrial revolution. As the steam engine and various mechanical devices spread throughout society, the tax of physical labor started to shrink. Work was still hard, but now machines were take over a lot of the physical work.

At first, people worked long hours in harsh conditions with the machines but as labor laws improved daily life became more flexible and filled with free time and other resources. Some of these resources were spent supporting the athletes who were performers in the arts and entertainment professions. These artists trained their body to perform at very high levels which amazed the labor intensive worker who did not pursue such athletic qualities. As interest in athletic performance grew some people took an interest in developing some of those capabilities as a hobby.

Sensing an entrepreneurial opportunity, the athletic performers realized they could sell products promising their levels of physical ability to the ordinary individual whose strength and fitness had been on the decline because of an increasingly sedentary lifestyle. These business minded performers sparked a new trend that encouraged people to be fit for the joy of it. Physical exercise was starting to become a casual pastime.

Even though fitness was becoming a niche hobby, most people still regarded the notion of working out as a usual thing to do. I even remember growing up with older adults telling me I was a crazy to go out for a run or lift weights just for the sake of fitness. "If you want exercise, go chop firewood or help the farmer load in his hay" they would tell me.

Some health experts even used to believed exercise was a dangerous endeavor. Doctors and health experts looked at hard physical cause as counterproductive towards health and well-being. People used to fear a condition known as "athlete's heart"

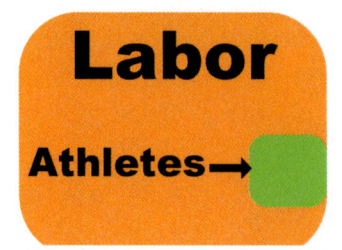

People learned how to condition their body to excel in specialized pursuits.

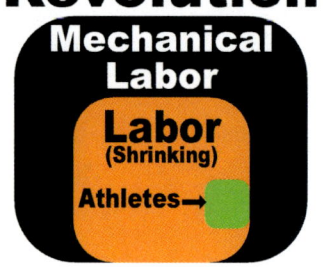

Machines start to remove the physical stress from work.

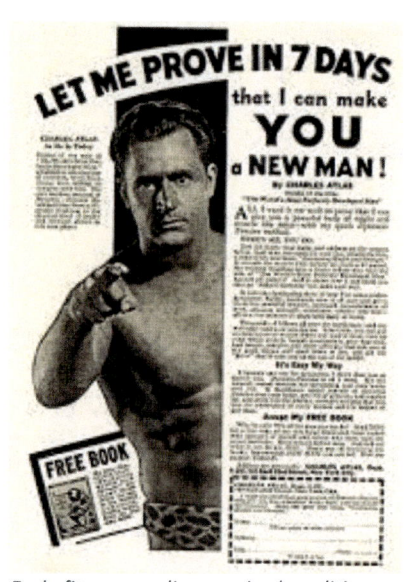

Early fitness media promised qualities industrial workers started to lack, like strength and toughness.

which is now commonly referred to as a heart attack.

So even until as recently as a generation ago, exercise and conditioning mostly fell within the scope of those who condition their body by trade or as a quirky hobby within a narrow subculture of society. It was very similar to how people only used computers for a job or an unusual hobby back when I was a kid. For exercise and physical conditioning to take society by storm, there needed to be a new revolution to bring the interest of fitness to the masses.

One of the most instrumental people in making this transformation happen was a man by the name of Bob Hoffman who founded the York Barbell Company in 1932. The York Barbell Co. created home study courses, sold home exercise equipment, made nutritional products, published magazines and even put on fitness competitions. Bob's influence reached a couple of brothers from Montreal Canada named Joe and Ben Weider. Joe and Ben set up a company that was similar to York Barbell. They were also selling equipment, supplements and holding fitness competitions, but their primary business was writing and producing magazines and periodicals. It was through their publishing empire the Weider brothers built one of the biggest philosophical fitness revolutions in modern society. That revolution became known as bodybuilding.

On the surface, Bob Hoffman and the Weiders were both in the business of selling fitness products, but their approach took very different paths. Whereas Bob Hoffman sold to the athletically minded individual, the Weiders began to focus more on using fitness as a means to alter the appearance of the body. Their competitions didn't involve much of the weightlifting and athletic events. Instead, they focused on how the body looked and appeared before a panel of judges. Whereas Bob Hoffman's focus may be on how to lift more weight or improve the ability to run, the Weider publications promised bigger arms, sleeker legs, and sex appeal.

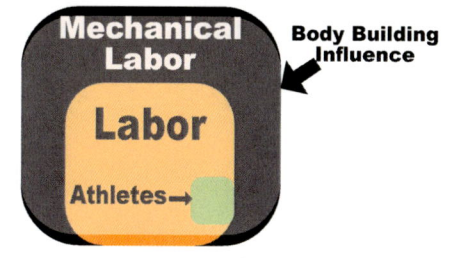

The body building philosophy takes over the world.

Here, at last, was an enticing reason for almost anyone to exercise and adopt a healthy lifestyle. Even if someone had no practical need to lift a lot of weight or run a fast race they still wanted to look good and feel attractive. By emphasizing the visual benefits of fitness, the bodybuilding philosophy blew down barriers that initially held back a widespread appreciation for exercise.

There were other reasons why the notion of bodybuilding grew to such popularity. First, it found fertile ground at a time when mass media was showcasing an ideal physical image in movies and magazines. American culture was becoming more open about showing skin and freedom of expressing the human body. Within a few short decades, a healthy and fit body became as much of a status symbol as a mansion or a luxury sports car. Having a healthy looking body meant you were a disciplined hard worker, and you possessed self-confidence. It also meant you had the lifestyle resources to make such physical changes happen. It no longer mattered if you were not a competitive athlete or needed to stay in shape to earn a paycheck. Being fit, or at least looking fit, was a sign of social status and sex appeal.

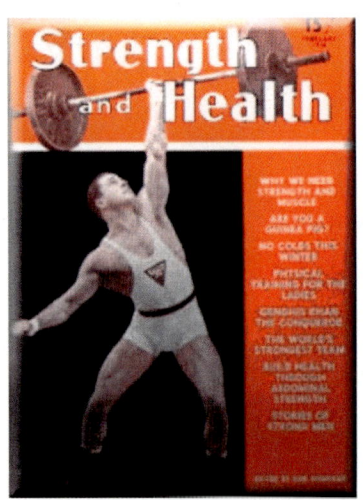

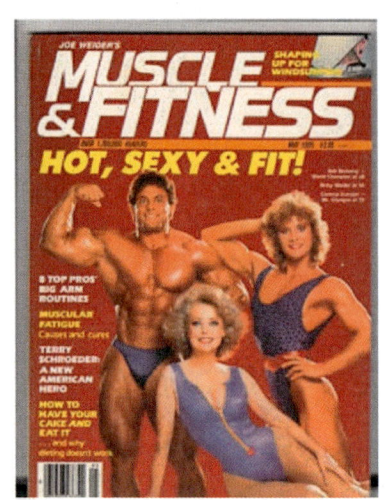

Older fitness media was more about developing health and strength. The newer body building media leaned towards developing an appearance.

The bodybuilding influence grew to include everyone. While the actual sport of bodybuilding may have initially focused on traditionally masculine pursuits like bigger muscles, it quickly spilled over into more widely accepted markets such as body sculpting or shaping. Body building also transcended various social divisions. Everyone wanted to look fit and healthy. The appeal of looking better transcended race, gender, religion, and tax bracket.

The bodybuilding revolution has continued to influence our views on diet and exercise right into our modern fitness culture. Walk into any gym and you'll find equipment born from a time when people targeted an area of the body to shape it as they wish. Fitness magazines promising health and vitality still entice us with sexy cover models and headlines promoting ways to shrink, sculpt, grow and chisel the body.

YouTube videos promising to show you how to cure muscle imbalances rack up a fraction of the views of a video with a thumbnail of ripped abdominals and a title promising a sexy physique. Even though the idea of functional training and becoming a weekend warrior has recently become more popular, people are still voting with their dollars for methods that promise shape and sex appeal over function and capability.

The mixed blessing of body building

The bodybuilding revolution has done beautiful things for spreading the value of a healthy diet and exercise. Gyms and associated fitness businesses have proliferated over the past half century. More people are practicing healthy habits than ever before.

The downside is that a lot of what has "sold" people on fitness is the shaky premise that getting in shape is associated with a positive change in the appearance of their body. All through human history training has been about building a stronger, faster and more capable body. The idea of training for the sake of shaping the body is largely a product of our imagination. It's a marketing strategy born from focus groups and modern appeal. Altering the shape of the body is not a bad or unhealthy pursuit, but it's not a high priority for Mother Nature.

You may now be thinking "Matt, you're crazy. What about the fact that people do change their body through diet and exercise?"

I'm not saying that working out and eating well won't change how you look. I'm saying there isn't as a stable connection between your physical ability and appearance as we've all been lead to believe. Evidence of this is everywhere. Walk into any gym or ask anyone who's adopted a regular exercise routine and you're guaranteed to find someone who became stronger and more capable of doing that workout. Someone who could hardly run 100 yards when they started can reliably be capable of running a 5K within a few months. The teenager who could hardly do five pushups will undoubtedly be able to do over 50 after following a pushup routine all summer. Ask the body to endure a new stressful function and you'll spark physiological change to better handle that stress 100% of the time. However, the results are less predictable if you ask that runner if they are losing weight, or if the teen has added inches to his arms.

How did our expectations get so far off track?

While fitness can make some change in your physical appearance, the speed and degree of these changes have become warped due to various factors. One of these is the marketing hype and promotion of inflated promises regarding just how much change is possible through using relatively weak products. Most of these products are cheap and easy to use making them easy to sell, but they are a small influence towards fulfilling a root cause. Just consider any cheap piece of fitness equipment sold through an infomercial. Chances are the "Ab Smasher 3000" won't do much to influence the appearance of your abs. It's cheap and easy to use, but the claim that it will "tone your core" is nothing more than empty hype.

Over time, these weak products have over promised and under delivered on those promises. Nevertheless, the hype has subconsciously taught people that the right diet or exercise program can directly make them look very different. Even though that ab training gadget wouldn't do much for you, the sexy models in the commercial still convey the idea that doing the right kind of training will make you look like them.

There is a host of other influences that are stretching the fragile link between fitness and physical appearance. Steroids and custom drug programs that directly change how the body looks are becoming more sophisticated and widespread. Plastic surgery and graphic design programs can further alter the reality of how much the body can change.

It's easy to see why these practices might be perceived as a form of cheating or deception. To maintain a clean image, individuals often practice these methods in secret while showcasing the effects under a spotlight or camera. To make sense of such unnatural changes, the people showing off their results attribute their new look to more acceptable methods. The body builder on steroids credits his split routine and the protein shake he endorses. The movie star who got plastic surgery and had a Photo Shopped magazine cover credits the latest yoga trend and their organic kale smoothie. While these more acceptable habits are certainly an influence, they have a much smaller impact compared to the underground habits practiced behind the camera. The result is those who don't suspect the celebrity is practicing these habits believe it's all down to a few simple diet and exercise habits.

Reality TV shows displaying radical physical transformations are also distorting our perception of what is possible. While these shows do use diet and exercise as a primary method for physical changes, they are another example of just how limited fitness can be towards improving the appearance of the body. In many of these shows, contestants devote their entire life towards little more than eating and exercising for the sake of changing their shape. In some cases, they remove every influence of their old lifestyle as they live at a secluded location where trainers and coaches have complete control over their life. These shows are an extreme example of how much the human body can change when someone is willing to spend every bit of their lifestyle resources towards a physical change. While these stories can be inspiring, it's important to understand that these transformations are taking place under very extreme conditions. The effects of diet and exercise can finally take credit, but to bring about significant changes, people need to go to extremes to make them happen.

We are currently riding a tidal wave of inflated beliefs that eating the right vegetables and working out a certain way will directly, and substantially, improve how your body will look. This notion has some truth to it, but it's been blown so far out of proportion that now people wonder why their body doesn't look much different from one week to the next even though they adopt a few diet and exercise habits.

Now the good news; your body *can* change its size and shape

So now that I've harped on the idea that the body doesn't have to make significant changes in appearance due to specific fitness habits, it's now time for some good news. The good news is you *can* alter the shape and appearance of your body to at least some degree. It's just that those ways never depend on a particular exercise or dietary program. These changes are also much more general than what you may read in the magazines. Let's first get into the cause of shaping the body and then explore the ways it can and can't change how you look.

The root cause of body shaping/sculpting /building

The first thing is to recognize that all forms of bodybuilding or body sculpting use the same two basic physiological changes. Our fitness culture loves to dream up different types of body shaping goals from sculpting, toning, bulking, building and even lengthening. These various goals are created to make fitness more individualized and complicated. It makes it easier to make different programs and products to convince the consumer they need very specific products to reach their objectives. Even though these products may claim to help different types of individuals, the actual process from one to the next is often the same. Shaping the human body does not require a specialized routine or program. In fact, when it comes to improving your appearance through fitness there are only two things you need to consider:

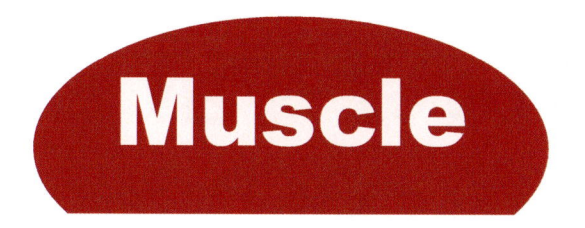

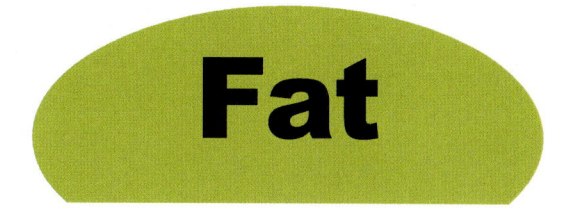

Muscle **Fat**

Almost all significant changes in the shape of your body are due to changing your fat mass or changing your muscle mass. Often it's a combination of the two. Everyone from the champion bodybuilder to the middle age executive who only wants to "look athletic" is manipulating the amount of the same two tissues on their body. The only difference is the degree of those changes.

It gets even simpler than that. All body shaping goals boil down to either decrease the amount of fat on their body or increase the amount of muscle, or a combination of the two. So it doesn't matter if you want to sculpt, tone up, bulk up, become massive or slim down. Pretty much everybody's playing the less-fat-and-more-muscle game.

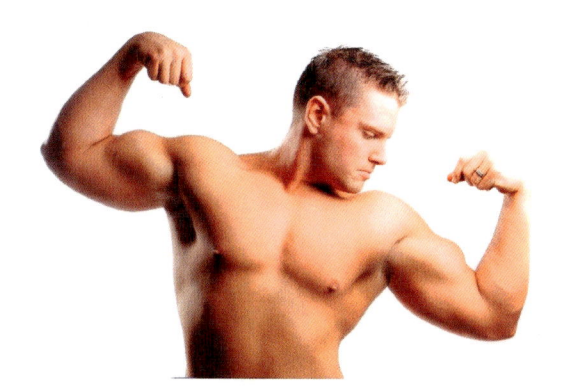

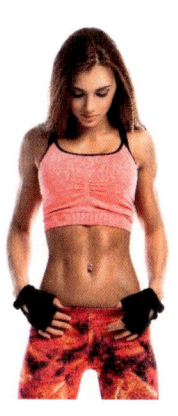

Despite the obvious differences, both of these fitness models have obtained their physique through adding muscle and decreasing fat mass.

What about water weight?

Water is yet another influence in the size and shape of your body. However, water is usually a somewhat transient factor which can change very quickly from day to day and even hour to hour. Manipulating water volume within the body is a concern for those who are looking to fine tune their appearance for a competition or event. It's not usually something that will have a drastic effect if the amount of muscle and fat are significant influences in how you want to look.

How realistic are fat and muscle changes?

The other thing about fat and muscle is they both influence the shape of your body in one of two ways. They both grow and they both shrink.

How Muscle & Fat Change in Appearance

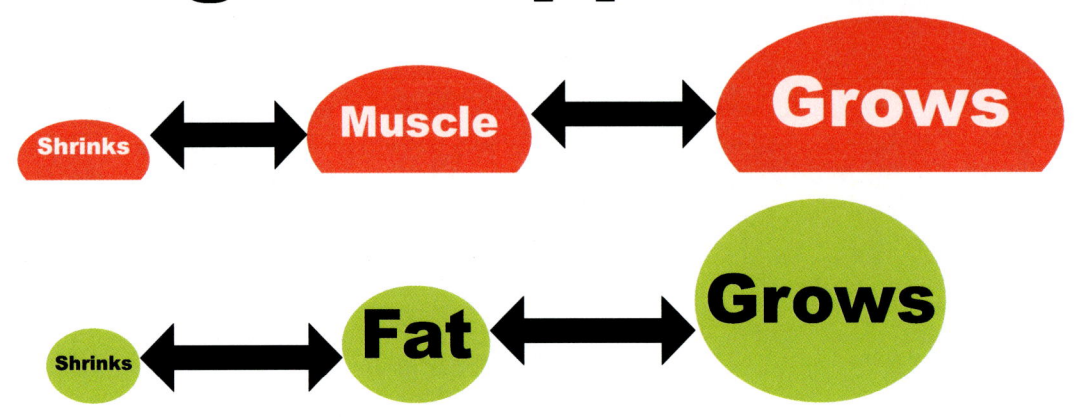

Both muscle and fat change your appearance through either growing or shrinking.

Once again, our fitness culture will present you with different methods as if you can modify the shape of these two tissues with some unnecessary programs or methods. But at the end of the day, all changes to your appearance come from muscle and fat tissue either growing or shrinking. Even though both fat and muscle grow or shrink, there are some differences between the two tissues regarding just how they can influence your physical appearance.

You can target muscles, but not fat

The cool thing about fat is you change the amount of it over your entire body at once. You can't selectively choose where you can lose or add body fat. While this may seem like a bad thing, it's actually a good thing.

Imagine if there was a program that allowed you to target fat loss in one particular area, like your belly. If that were the case, you would have to use lifestyle resources to lose fat in just that one area. Once that section of your body was lean, you would then need to use even more diet and exercise practices to lose the fat in your legs or arms. The additional program would take up even more resources as you would have to maintain the fat loss in the first area while working in the other areas. Thankfully you don't have to use many different exercises or dietary methods since you shed fat over your entire body at once.

I like to think of fat loss kind of like draining a swimming pool. The design of the swimming pool means that certain areas of the pool have deeper water than others. You can remove some of the water from the pool, but the water level drops over the entire pool at once. The deeper areas will always remain deeper than the shallower areas no matter how much water you take out. Your body is the same way. You cannot cause a deeper fat zone to become a shallow area and vice versa. No matter how lean you get, there will always be a noticeably larger amount of fat in the areas you naturally have more fat.

Unlike fat, muscle is a tissue you can target through various exercises. There are hundreds of different exercises you can do for any major muscle group. Even the simple push up has more variations than you would ever need over an entire lifetime. You can grow some muscles more while other muscles are neglected and remain small.

While you can target a muscle you can't change its shape

It's a myth that your muscles can change their shape. Muscle is just like fat in the way it either grows or shrinks. It cannot radically change its form or appearance beyond those two options. If one of your muscles is relatively narrow and long, it will always remain long and narrow no matter what you do. If it's round and short, it will stay that way too.

The volume of fat is often easier to change than the volume of muscle

Some supplement advertisements claim the human body will quickly and easily build massive amounts of muscle, but this is rarely the case. The average person can pack on 50 or 60 pounds of additional fat, but it's very hard for most folks to add even 15 or 20 pounds of muscle. That's not to say adding even a few pounds of muscle won't make a noticeable difference. Adding even a little extra muscle will have a very noticeable influence towards how your body looks and feels.

Both fat and muscle size is affected by how many cells you start with

Both fat and muscle grow and shrink by enlarging the size of your existing cells. Naturally, someone who has more fat cells will tend to have higher fat levels than someone who has a lower number of fat cells. The same goes for muscle growth. Someone who starts off with a lot of muscle cells will have the potential to get much bigger than someone who's comparatively small.

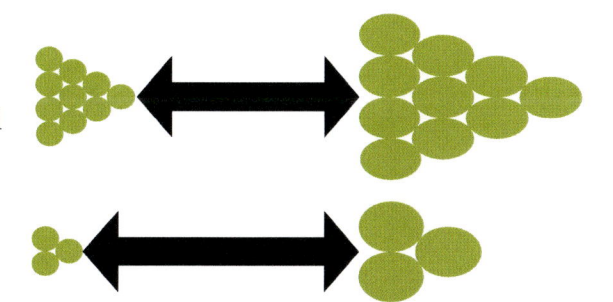

Your potential to change both fat and muscle mass depends on how many cells you have.

Both fat and muscle break down as a default

The default setting of your physique is to break down over time. Your body is always trying to shed as much muscle and fat as possible. The degree you fulfill the cause of fat and muscle is what supports the level you have. Even as you read this, your body is trying to rid itself of both your muscle and body fat. While this might seem obvious as far as muscle is concerned, it's sometimes hard to imagine that's the case with body fat. If anything it's easier to believe the body will get fatter all on its own.

Even traditional fitness science seems to support this idea. Many theories claim humans have survived harsh times by storing fat and shedding muscle. I take exception to this idea because it gives off this very demoralizing view that we have evolved to be fat, weak and lazy and getting in shape is going against our nature. What a bunch of baloney! The human body didn't change to be unfit any more than it evolved to breathe underwater. Sure people can become out of shape, but it's through modern intervention rather than the curse of evolution. The only reason why we have been able to survive is that our body can become more agile, mobile and active. We can fight, run, climb, jump, lift, throw and do any number of athletic activities. We can even adapt to a wide range of climates with various food sources. Humans live everywhere from the tundra to the tropical forest. The only way this is even possible is because our bodies are highly adaptable and can become stronger.

Muscle is also a heck of a lot more important towards your survival than fat. As I mentioned in the cause of muscle chapter, muscle is critical towards your overall health, fitness and performance. Being able to build, hunt, fight, and travel depend highly on how strong you are. Even in today's modern society the soft and weak don't thrive and live as long as those who are stronger. If being weak makes life harder today it would have made it almost impossible back then. It is true that the human body evolved to store fat, but it has also evolved to burn fat as well. Accumulating a storage tank of fuel that's tough to burn leaves you with little evolutionary advantage. It makes you slower and less agile. The fatter you are, the more resources you need to maintain your size and back then resources were a lot harder to acquire. There's no question about it; humans have evolved to be healthy and fit.

So why is building muscle and burning fat so difficult?

It mainly boils down to personal habits and the environment. Some folks have the habit of always ordering the largest size soda at the drive through because it's a "better value" while insisting they cannot miss their favorite TV programs. Other people can't help but make a healthy meal for dinner, and they feel restless if they sit still for more than 30 minutes. Some of these habits have become entrenched in the person's life through years, even decades, of daily repetition. They become so automatic the person is not even aware of how those habits are influencing their root causes. At that point, the outcome feels automatic, almost effortless.

The different practices would be "unnatural" if those two people switched places. The important lesson is that you're not built to assume any state of fitness automatically. You can set your internal autopilot on fat-and-weak mode just as much as you can set it on lean-and-strong mode. It all boils down to the habits you choose that influence your root causes as opposed to some evolutionary traits you have no control over.

Personal influences of your muscle building potential

Everyone has the potential to shed fat and build muscle regardless of age, genetics or lifestyle. Still, some folks have more potential to alter their fat and muscle levels than others. Some will build muscle easier while other people may find it simpler to pack on fat. While no one has a permanently set body size, it is important to recognize some of the personal factors that can influence your potential.

Factors in muscle building

The first of these influences is your gender. The hormones within the body play an enormously influential role in your potential to build muscle, and typically the males have more of these hormones, primarily testosterone.

The second significant influence is age. People never lose the ability to build muscle and grow stronger; however, the peak years for muscle growth are typical between the later stages of adolescence and into middle age. As you age, the speed of growth and the total amount of muscle you can grow slightly decreases each year.

The third major influence is how much of your genetic potential you have used up through years of training. While it's very rare for someone to reach the limits of their genetic potential, it does become harder to progress as you grow. This is Precisely why someone new to training may find they can build muscle much easier than someone who has been training for many years.

The last thing to consider is your overall genetic build. Just like with body fat, muscle cells increase in size rather than number. Someone who has more muscle cells to start with has a greater chance of growing more muscle volume.

With these factors in mind, it's possible to see why some people are at more of an advantage to build muscle than others. If I wanted to train someone with the intention of building as much muscle mass as possible, my choice would be for a 25-year-old male who already had a lot of muscle on their frame but has never done any strength training.

The individual with a far lower chance of building a lot of muscle would probably fit the profile of a 60-year-old petite female who has been doing strength training for the past 20 years. Even if I gave the same program to these two individuals both would stand a good chance of becoming bigger and stronger but the younger male who had never lifted weights before would be sure to put on a lot more muscle.

No, you can't have the same body as someone else

It's physically impossible for your body to look like someone else. You can't alter your body to resemble someone you see in a magazine or a movie. If you lose a lot of body fat you won't look like a French supermodel; you'll look like a leaner version of yourself. You can't look like Arnold Schwarzenegger no matter how much muscle put on your frame. You'll simply have a bigger and more muscular version of the body you have right now. I'm not bringing this up to discourage you but to set your mind free from unrealistic expectations. Besides, the world doesn't want another Arnold Schwarzenegger or Kate Moss. People want to see the unique physical traits that you and only you can bring to the world.

So to sum it all up, changing the shape of your body is controlled by the cause of the balance between your fat and muscle levels. Both fat and muscle change through an increase or decrease in volume and while you can target which muscles get bigger or smaller, fat levels change over the body as a whole. How much you can improve your fat and muscle levels is influenced by your genetics and overall build as well as other factors such as age and training experience. You'll always have the body you have now, but you can modify in a couple of ways.

So how do you grow or shrink your body?

Regardless of what your physique shaping goals are, you're trying to shrink certain areas through a reduction of body fat while building or sculpting other areas through building muscle.
We have already covered how calorie balance is the cause controlling the amount of fat on your body, so that's one-half of the equation. Now let's dive into the cause of what makes your muscle change in size.

The cause of muscle growth

I purposely left out the cause of muscle growth from the cause of muscle chapter so I could discuss it in further detail here. One of the biggest reasons is because the adaptation to almost all muscular training is to condition *capability*, not appearance. Also, understanding the S.A.I.D principle is critical towards influencing the cause of muscle growth.

What causes muscle growth?

Just like growing or shrinking a fat cell, the reason for muscle growth is also a balance between two influences with each being of equal importance. Just as calories in vs. calories out is the cause of changing your fat levels, your muscle levels change due to the balance between the mechanical stress a muscle endures and its ability to recover from that stress.

Just as with calorie balance, It's the *relationship* between stress and recovery that determines what condition your muscles are in. A lot of stress requires a lot of recovery. A little bit of physical stress needs a little recovery and so on. Just as no food or activity alone can control how much fat you have, no exercise or food can be solely responsible for causing your muscles to grow.

How do you use the stress/ recovery balance to grow muscle?

Before I get too much into the cause of muscle growth, it's key to understand that science is still trying to figure out exactly what causes muscle growth. Some research points to cellular damage, while some suggest it's a hormonal change or maybe even something to do with your nervous system. At this stage in my understanding, I believe there are many factors to consider which may all play a part so I'm presenting a perspective here that I think should leave you well covered.

Just like with calorie balance, the stress and recovery balance isn't something you need to create. It's already happening to you every day. Even if you stand up and walk to the fridge, you're using your, muscles to accomplish that activity. Of course only standing and walking across the room uses little energy and it doesn't create that much demand for physical capability. Still, even if the demand is weak, it is still there and maintaining at least some level of muscular size and strength. When you create a mechanical stress in muscle, you're directly telling your body that it needs to maintain the capability to do that activity.

If you want to improve and grow your muscles, then you must demand even more energy use from your muscle. When you do this, something very cool happens. As always, your body will recover through replacing that chemical energy but since you triggered a bit more stress than it was expecting your body overcompensates by putting a tiny bit more "juice" into the muscle fibers than you initially used. When this happens, your muscles become ever so slightly bigger through super-compensation. When this cycle repeats itself, those little bits of super compensation build up to some pretty impressive muscle growth over time. Of course the opposite can happen as well. If the stress on a muscle decreases, the recovery process doesn't have to put back quite as much chemical energy and the muscle shrinks.

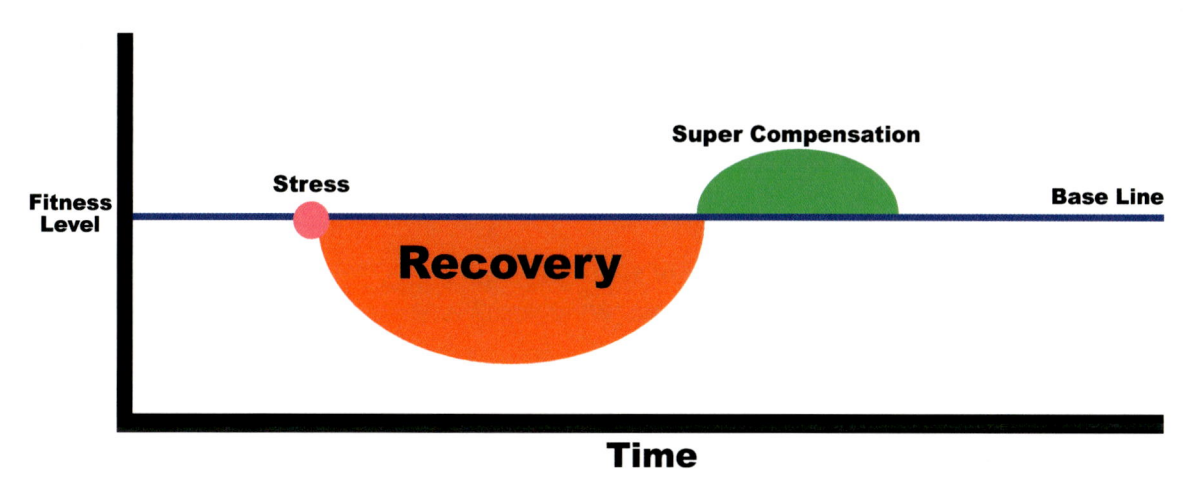

A single round of the stress and recovery cycle with a brief period of super compensation.

The balance between stress and recovery has many influences on each side. Here are a few of the biggest influences to keep in mind.

1. **Mechanical stress is from all physical activity, not just exercise**

Mechanical stress includes any and all voluntary muscle contraction. It's not just exercise or strength training. Any time your brain instructs your muscle fibers to contract some of that

73

chemical energy is used up regardless of what you are doing. It doesn't have to be within the confines of a workout or through the utilization of a particular piece of equipment.

A good example of this is how astronauts lose muscle mass when they spend time in a zero gravity environment. Even though you may not be working out here on earth, just walking around, with gravity pulling you downwards, causes some stress on your muscles which helps maintain their size and strength. Astronauts are not subject to this pressure in zero gravity so their muscle strength and size can diminish at an astonishing rate.

2. Only your brain can control muscular stress

Even though lifting something heavy is often credited with creating mechanical stress, it's your brain that is responsible for the tension in your muscle. This is where that S.A.I.D principle comes into play when it comes to building muscle. Lifting a weight or doing an exercise is just an influence on the stress a muscle is under. Ultimately it's your brain that controls what muscles are being used and to what degree they are contracting while doing the activity. This is why it's critical to improve your mental control over the tension in your muscles. The more you can control the tension in your muscles, the more mechanical stress there will be on the muscle fibers.

You can try this out for yourself the next time you stand up and walk. As you make your strides, try to concentrate on using your hamstrings to pull the front leg backward. You don't have actually to walk any differently, just focus on using the muscles in the back of your legs a little more to propel you forwards. Within a few steps, you'll notice that your legs feel a bit different as your brain uses a slightly different muscle activation pattern to walk. So even though you may be walking the same way, your brain has slightly altered the motor unit activation pattern and thus the stress on your muscles.

3. All exercises involves some degree of strength training

Our fitness culture loves to draw imaginary lines dividing training methods into groups such as some exercises are for strength, some are for endurance and so on. At the root, any activity that involves muscle contraction is strength training. Walking requires the power in your legs to move you forward and to hold your body up. Stretching in Yoga requires tension to hold a pose and to move from one position to another. Even "cardio" like using an elliptical requires the strength of the legs to move the pedals back and forth. So really, any and all forms of exercise are strength training to at least some degree.

4. Challenge your muscle to build muscle

Remember, the S.A.I.D principle states you gain that which you challenge. So if you want to gain muscle, you must test your muscle. This is where the idea of "muscle building exercises" or workouts come into play. Even though walking does place some mechanical stress on your leg muscles, the potential to build up those muscles is limited by how much you can challenge your muscles by walking. If you were an astronaut returning from 6 months in space walking would provide plenty of mechanical stress, and it would stimulate some muscle growth.

However, for someone who walks around most of the day, it's not going to build any more muscle. This is why you need to progressively challenge your muscles and their ability to contract. There are many ways you can do this. You can use a weight machine or a heavy object as you use your leg muscles. You can also do activities that require more work from your legs like running or hiking up a hill.

5. Time under tension

Time and tension are the two variables you have at your disposal to deplete the chemical energy within your muscle cells. These two variables are a bit in conflict with one another. If you can do an exercise for an extended period (like walking for 3 hours), chances, are the tension on the muscles is pretty small. On the other hand, you can do something that's very intense, like doing squats on one leg, but you won't be able to do it for very long.

I'm often asked if it's better to do a lot of reps with a light resistance or if it's better to do very few reps with heavy resistance. I say do both! Try to do a lot of reps with a lot of resistance. You might think that's impossible, but that's precisely the point. Remember, your body only cares about what it can *do*. The only way you can convince it to make any change is to try to do something that is just outside of what it considers a normal function. It doesn't matter if you can do a lot of resistance for low reps or light resistance for high reps. If either is within the range of what you can comfortably do your body won't have much reason to change beyond where you are now.

A million different programs can promise to help you build muscle, but here is the simplest and the most reliable way to exercise for muscle growth. Step 1) Select an activity that requires your mind to create a mental signal that places tension within the muscles you want to build. Step 2) Select a degree of difficulty that allows a consistent and reliable level of tension within the muscles you want to work. Step 3) Keep the amount of tension the same as you strive to do the exercise for a greater amount of time, preferably without stopping. Step 4) Once you can comfortably perform the exercise for a modest amount of time, increase the difficulty, so you're now creating more tension in the muscle. When you do this the amount of time, you can do that exercise will drop. From there you build up the amount of time you can do with the new level of tension, and you repeat the entire process.

It's a simple method, and it works. The most reliable way to build muscle is to train your muscles to be able to handle more tension for a longer period of time. Not only does it improve the capability to do the exercise, but it also builds some serious muscle as well.

So there you have it, pretty much every muscle building tip, trick, and article broken down into a few pages. Almost everything and anything regarding your training should strive for increasing the amount of tension on a muscle or the amount of time it can endure a given amount of tension. Everything else just details.

Now that we've covered the stress half of the muscle building cycle let us explore the recovery side of the balance. For the most part, recovery is any activity allows your body to rest and rebuild itself in preparation for the next stressful event or workout. Recovery can include, but is not limited to, your sleep, recreation, diet, massage, and relaxation both physically and mentally. When it comes to the physical recovery of your muscles two of the biggest influences are sleep and nutrition. I cover the cause of healthy eating in the next chapter but for now, the most basic rules of healthy eating will suit you just fine. These include the following:

1. **Keep your meals consistent**

Consistency is the foundation of all success with both diet and exercise. When it comes to healthy eating, try to keep what you eat, when you eat and how much you eat relatively consistent on a weekly basis. You don't have to eat the same meal every day at the same time, but keeping some general consistency makes it much easier to monitor and control how well you can recover in between workouts. If your diet consists of nothing but organic salad greens one day and a lot of junk food the next your body will have a much harder time adapting to both your diet and your workouts.

2. **Try to stick to natural foods as much as possible**

As I like to say, if you want to grow you need to eat things that once grew as well. Generally speaking, foods that come from a farm will help you recover faster than foods from a box or a bottle. This also goes for supplements. Nothing in a pill or powder will be as helpful for your recovery as something that grew out of the dirt or walked around.

3. **Follow your hunger and listen to your body**

Sometimes recovery requires a little more food. Other times it may require a little less. Listen to your body and learn to trust it. Most of the time it knows what's best for you.

The importance of sleep

I've learned the biggest limiting influence in many people's recovery is a lack of sleep. Even if someone's diet is on point and their workouts are fantastic, it's their sleep that still holds them back. Unfortunately, honoring sleep is sometimes seen as a weakness. Many people subscribe to the idea that you should keep your nose to the grindstone and forsake sleep in the name of work or productivity. I do not agree with this idea at all. No matter how strong or tough you are, you're severely handicapping yourself if you regularly test how little sleep you can get by on. It's just like back in the day when coaches used to make athletes practice without water under the mistaken belief it would toughen them up. Now we know such a practice does nothing but limit performance and put people's health at risk. Going with little sleep does the same thing.

Thankfully science is finally catching onto the idea that sleep is critical towards your health and fitness. Lack of sleep influences a host of ills ranging from hormone regulation, appetite control,

weight gain, blood sugar regulation, mood, productivity, muscle growth and cognitive performance. In short, sleep does both your body and mind right.
Just like with diet, healthy sleep habits are pretty basic.

1. Try to maintain consistent times when you go to bed and wake up in the morning

Widely varying sleep patterns make it difficult for both body and mind to find sure footing on a daily basis.

2. Have the wind-down routine an hour or so before going to sleep

Taking a hot bath or shower and reading something before bed can help your body and mind slow down and be ready for sleep.

3. Avoid blue light screens before bed

Staring at a bright screen before going to bed just tells your mind that you need to stay awake and alert. Trust me; there isn't anything on social media or on your favorite websites that can wait until morning. The last thing you want is to watch a video or read a news story that's designed to get you all wound up before you go to sleep.

Devices like E-readers with E-ink displays are fine. It's the bright backlit screens which emit blue light that can cause sleep disruption. If you must work on a computer or smartphone right before bed, see if you can find a blue light filter for the screen.

4. You want your sleep to be uninterrupted through the whole night

Avoid alcoholic drinks within an hour or so of going to bed. After all, ensure you don't have to wake up and go to the bathroom after falling asleep. Keep as much light out of the room as possible.

You want to avoid anything that's very stimulating such as music, caffeine, or video shortly before going to bed. It was always said that New York City was the city that never slept, but now the electronic age has made every household the home that never sleeps. Just like your workout and your healthy diet, the world will try to squeeze a good night's sleep from your life if you let it. Defend your ability to get a good night's sleep just as you would fight for your right to eat well and exercise.

Recovery is more than just physical rest

Mental stress can build up just as much as physical stress. Your mind needs to rest just as much as your body does. It's not healthy to always be stressed about being productive 24/7. Your body will follow your mind so even if your body is fresh it will feel exhausted if your mind is fried. This is why mental recovery is just as important to your muscle building efforts as physical rehabilitation.

Once again, this is sometimes seen as a weakness. You're not supposed to take a break and kick back except for maybe on Saturday night or an annual vacation. Working and keeping your nose to the grindstone is a sign that you're tough and not a wimp. People even brag about how much they sacrifice to keep mentally grinding away. If one guy works 12 hours a day, another will try to one-up him by saying he works seven days a week and so on. Usually, this goes hand in hand with how little sleep they can "get by on."

Fitness and life, in general, is not a game where the person who can withstand the most stress and hardship wins. If anything, you want to make this whole fitness thing as easy as possible, that's the whole point of Fitness Independence. When you make things needlessly difficult and stressful, all you do is hold yourself back. You end up spending twice the effort to get half as much done. Meanwhile the "lazy wimps" find ways to get twice as much done with half the effort.

The more resources you spend doing unnecessary work, the less you have left over to do what matters most. You can brag about working 16 hours and driving yourself into the ground with harsh diet and exercise routines, but Mother Nature doesn't give a damn about how hard you can push yourself. All she cares about, and subsequently rewards, is what you can get done and how well you can do it. If you can do that with a 30-minute workout and a modest diet, then you win. Fulfilling the same cause with twice the work doesn't make you tougher or more bad ass. It makes you less efficient, and you're wasting resources you could spend towards other priorities in life.

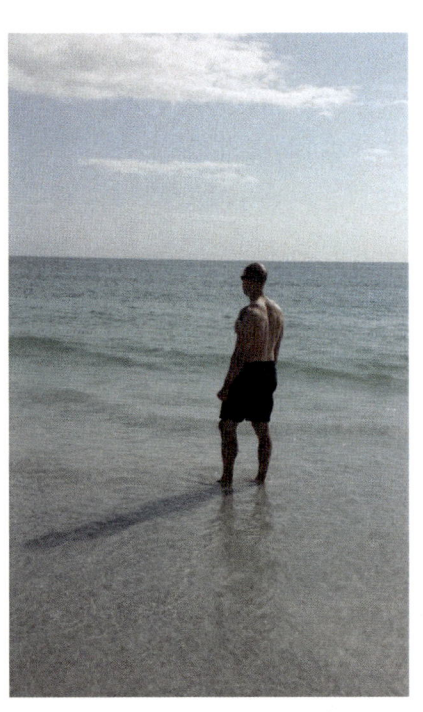

The world isn't such a bad place if you can just manage to get out into it.

So have fun every day, not just on Saturday night. Hang out with your friends, even if it's just out on your front porch while watching the sunset. I promise it's a lot more beneficial to your mind than watching late night TV or scrolling through your social media feed for the 15th time. Play games, do anything that can inspire a little creativity or competition. If nothing else, just get outside and let the natural world finally get between you and your smartphone. Sometimes the best thing you can do for your mind is to stop worrying and let the world keep on spinning while knowing that it's not all on your shoulders.

Both mental and physical recovery is essential. They are not a luxury. When your recovery is better, you come back to your workout with more energy and power than you had before due to that super compensation. It's that very recovery that makes you more fit over time.
If you come back to your workout, and you're not 1% better than before you won't be able to advance. You'll be stuck grinding away and doing the same work just to stay where you are.

Okay, so you've got the cause of what it takes to alter the shape of your body. Now let's further explore what this cause means to you and just how far you can take it.

Can you build muscle and burn fat at the same time?

People often ask me if it's possible to build muscle and lose fat at the same time, and the answer is a resounding YES! Not only is it possible, but it's even likely. To understand why remember that fat and muscle are two different tissues on your body, so they both have separate root causes. You can separately alter the fat and muscle mass just as you can do something with one hand and something else with the other.

The conventional idea is that muscle growth happens because you work the muscle and eat a lot. Fat loss happens because you eat less and move more, preferably with energy-draining exercise like cardio. From this perspective, it would seem that muscle and fat were in opposition of one another. How can you build muscle and burn fat if one requires you to eat a lot and the other requires you to eat less?

The answer is that eating a lot of food doesn't cause muscle growth. Yes, an inadequate diet can hold back muscle growth through slowing down your recovery, but eating by itself won't tell your muscles to grow bigger and stronger. Diet is merely an influence to the cause of both muscle and fat. Granted it's typically greater importance for fat levels than it is for muscle, but it's still just an influence nonetheless.

I fully admit that it's a lot harder to be in a negative calorie balance and still put enough tension on muscle for it to become stronger. It's much easier to recover when you're eating plenty of natural food, but just because it's harder to do something doesn't mean it's impossible. If the muscle work and recovery are there, then the muscle will grow even if you're in a negative calorie balance.

So yes, you can build muscle and lose fat at the same time. You also don't have to put on fat to build muscle. Getting fatter is no more a necessity for muscle building than holding your breath while walking in the rain. Some experts claim you have to be in a "caloric surplus" to build muscle. Again, this is a complete myth. If it were true at all, then our obesity epidemic would also have a correlation of strong, very muscular individuals.

The calorie surplus myth

A caloric surplus always results in a fat gain, and *never* muscle gain. The very definition of a surplus is having more than is needed. So if you're consuming more calories and you don't need them for anything (including muscle growth) they are either passed or stored as fat. It's impossible for a caloric surplus to build muscle. If you do eat more and it helps fuel your recovery and muscle growth, then it's not a surplus by the very fact that you can use those calories.

Also, what if you train hard, and you do need some additional calories to aid in your recovery, but you don't eat them for one reason or another? How on earth are you supposed to recover if you don't eat enough? Well, wouldn't it be great if your body had a storage tank of calories it could pull from during times when you don't eat enough? Of course, you see where I'm going with this. If you do need some additional calories to aid your recovery you have plenty of them readily available in your fat stores! So if you do need extra calories, don't worry. You're carrying them on you right now in your fat. You'll be burning fat to build muscle which is the reason why I say that not only can you burn fat and build muscle at the same time, but it may even be more likely to happen.

Why is the idea of eating a caloric surplus so attractive?

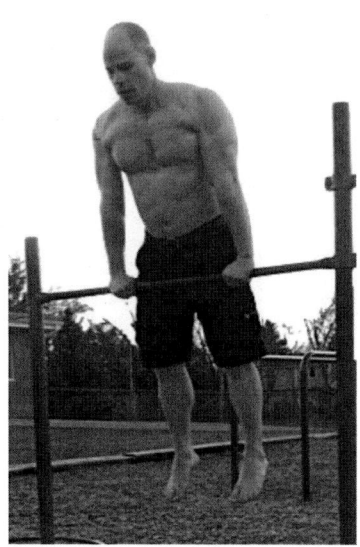

Building muscle is more about what you put into your training rather than what you put on your plate.

There are many reasons why people jump to the conclusion that you need to eat a lot to build muscle. One of the reasons is because it just seems logical. You're trying to add something to your body, so naturally, you're going to have to consume something extra. After all, you can't build something up without the raw materials, right?

Another reason is muscle building is big business, and much of it is from pills, shakes, bars, and other products you have to buy. The more the media claims you can't build muscle unless you consume enough of their product the easier it is to sell you stuff. Of course, you don't need any of these things to build muscle. Remember, muscle building, and fitness, in general, is a big business which is funny. Nothing humans have ever invented is required to build a healthy and fit body. We didn't create fitness, Mother Nature did. We're just trying to add some fancy toys and gadgets to add some flavor to the soup that was cooked up long before we even knew what soup even was.

Over the years I've watched as the business of supplements has grown to obscene levels. It used to be about selling protein powder you would consume after a workout a few times a week. Now there are products to consume in the morning, afternoon and night. There are products to consume before your workout, during your workout, and after your workout. None of this stuff is necessary to build muscle. Mother Nature set up the entire muscle building process, allowing people to grow all the muscle they would need long before this stuff came out.

Here in America, I'm part of the most overfed society on earth. It's one of the reasons why so many people are struggling to lose weight. Somehow I'm supposed to believe that the five egg breakfast burrito, the foot-long sandwich for lunch and the 16-ounce steak for dinner, plus all of those snacks isn't enough? Most folks eat more in a single meal than many people eat all day while muscle building companies are doing a magnificent job trying to convince them they should be buying and ingesting a lot of other products. Talk about selling sand to a man in the desert! Eating more to build muscle might be an issue if you find it a challenge to eat 3 square meals a day. Beyond that, you probably get enough through a sufficient breakfast, lunch, and dinner.

Another driving force behind the eat-to-build muscle idea is the professional athletes who have a much higher calorie and nutrition requirements than the average individual. The heavy training load these people undergo on a daily basis is far beyond what the dedicated exercise enthusiast experiences. Some of these athletes undertake more training in a day than most people do in a week or even a month! This sort of training creates a massive nutritional demand and supplements can make it easier to satisfy that need. After all, what seems more natural, slurping down a couple of protein shakes or taking the time to prepare and eat three extra meals?

As much as I like to believe I'm an active guy, my daily 60-minute workout is not that much of an influence to my nutritional needs. Even if I trained every day, that's only 7 hours of extra activity each week. It might seem like a lot, but compared to serious athletes it's not very much.

Also, don't forget the role drugs can play in creating more nutritional demand. Steroids can produce an unnatural level of muscle and a super speedy recovery. This abnormal development can create a dietary demand far above what most people need.

Lastly, there's the bodybuilding theory that you can "bulk" by force feeding yourself a lot and lifting aggressively to force muscle growth. Most of the time, this involves eating a lot more food and lifting heavier weights. The result is the person's weight goes up, and they get stronger in the gym. Many believe the extra weight and strength is proof they are packing on beef.

Unfortunately, this is not always the case. Gaining fat can make a person both look and feel bigger. It also makes the muscles feel bigger because some of the fat deposits reside in the muscle tissue itself. At the same time, aggressive lifting can cause an increase in strength, but this is mostly due to a greater use of motor units. At the end of the day, you have an individual who looks and feels bigger and is, in fact, stronger. Even though they have some more jiggle around their waist, they are told to accept that as a natural consequence of building muscle.

The hard truth is that muscle growth is usually a very slow process often taking months or even a year or two to notice any significant changes. This slow growth can make it difficult for people in the muscle building business to convince customers to keep using their products and services when there is a little noticeable difference from one week to the next. It's much easier, and quicker, to add fat and improve strength neurologically than it is to build muscle. You can add 20 pounds to yourself and feel much stronger within a couple of weeks. If I can convince you that it means you're building muscle, then you're much more likely to continue investing in what I'm selling.

The reality is that most folks, myself included, simply don't need all of that extra food and supplementation to build muscle. Even if your workouts are over an hour, you're probably not that much more active than someone who has a moderately active profession. I wouldn't tell a waitress or a doctor who's on their feet all day they need to eat a lot more because of their job. Why would I tell someone they need to eat a lot more because they hit the gym a few times a week?

You can see how all of this can create a perfect storm of influences telling you if you don't eat enough and ingest the right products then you can't build muscle. You have businesses trying to sell you products. You have professional athletes, both natural and on steroids, with a very high nutritional demand and you also have the very idea that you're trying to add something to your body. It all boils down to the idea that if you want to build muscle and be like the pros, then you had better chow down!

The real question isn't if a calorie surplus is necessary. By definition, a surplus is not something you need to have. The real issue is if you should eat more than you currently are if you want to build muscle. Unfortunately, that's not an answer I can supply for you. It would even be irresponsible of me even to try because, in all honesty, I don't know. There's no way I can know; there are just too many influences at work here. Influences I don't know about because it's your body and your life. Maybe you would be well off to add a tuna sandwich to your lunch pail, perhaps not. To help you figure it out though turn the page as we dive into the cause of a healthy diet.

7: The Cause of Healthy Eating

Before I discovered Fitness Independence, eating right was a constant source of both physical and mental stress. These days I consider diet one of the easiest aspects of my lifestyle. I hardly even have to think about it, let alone stress over how to eat right from one day to the next. Even though I'm spending a fraction of the effort, I'm far healthier, leaner, and stronger. I also have no problem maintaining my results without spending resources to stay up on the latest dietary theories and fads.

I learned about the cause of healthy eating through challenging the very idea of what it meant to eat properly. What I discovered was that some of the favorite messages about a healthy diet are counterproductive towards eating for the sake of health and wellbeing. While many of these ideas may not be that bad on their own, they all combined to create a perfect storm that can prevent you from fulfilling the cause of healthy eating.

The perfect storm of eating right

The first, and perhaps biggest reason why eating right is such a struggle is the almost universal acceptance that a healthy diet is incredibly important towards any fitness goal. Any expert will not think twice to tell you that diet is an important part of any fitness program regardless of what you're after.

The acceptance of the importance of diet has fueled the next idea that not only is nutrition important, but it's vital. Many experts even claim the lion's share of your success boils down to diet. Some say things like "90% of success is diet" and "You can't out-train a bad diet." Exaggerated claims like this raise the importance of what you eat to an unprecedented level.

Not only is diet super important towards improving your chance of getting in shape, but it's also supposedly super important in improving your entire quality of life. I've witnessed many minds travel down a slippery slope as they depend heavily on a diet to improve health and soon perceive food as a way to prevent other health issues ranging from performance at work and school to protection against seemingly random misfortunes like natural disasters. Because of this, almost everything in someone's life can be credited to, or even blamed for the condition of one's diet.

The high importance of eating right leads right into the next belief that eating right is a complicated science. Go to any bookstore and you'll find shelves filled with thick books on how to eat right, written by people who have dedicated their career towards figuring out the perfect diet. There are entire institutions, companies and organizations working around the clock in an attempt to solve the nutrition puzzle. Even asking a personal trainer what they recommend for a post workout snack will invite a lecture straight out of chemistry class.

Since nutrition is so complicated, it only makes sense to turn to the experts who obviously know a lot more about how to eat right. They are the ones doing the cutting edge research and spending the time trying to put the puzzle together. So obviously they know the best way to eat right.

Because the experts are the ones in the know, those who are not dedicated to studying nutrition shouldn't be trusted to figure out what to do on their own. Not only are you in the dark about how you should be eating, but you also can't even trust yourself to eat healthy if left to your choices. Many theories claim evolution has programmed you to crave and become addicted to foods that contain every unhealthy ingredient imaginable. To make matters worse, many food companies, who seemingly only care about profits, are trying to produce terrible foods that you supposedly can't help yourself from eating, and you'll endlessly gorge yourself until both your body and your quality of life are at risk of ruin.

You are your worst enemy and can't responsibly handle foods that are just as addictive and harmful as narcotics. Whatever you do, don't trust yourself to make sound food choices. Let the experts tell you what's best. The very best thing you can do is wage war with yourself on a daily basis. Denial and sacrifice are now your badges of honor. All of the stress and guilt that comes from preventing yourself from eating wrong is proof that you're doing a great job of fighting yourself and winning the battle. Remember, feeling miserable is a sign that you're adopting healthy habits.

The next step in this perfect storm is the lack of agreed upon rules when it comes to how to actually eat right. Some People believe you should avoid meat, while others say you need to eat a lot of meat but avoid grains. Some claim fruit is the best thing for you and others claim it's terrible. One expert gives a recommendation for how much protein you should eat while another claims that's far too much or too little. Everyone has their set of rules and theories on how you should eat right, and they all appear to contradict each other.

In an attempt to add credibility to their ideas, each expert comes to the table armed with very convincing proof why their way is best. First, they have a lot of scientific evidence built upon years of research and studies. This scientific data appeals to your desire for logical proof that their theory isn't just dreamed up out of nowhere. There's also the social proof that their theory works in the real world. Sports stars, celebrities and other high profile members of society give their endorsement claiming the diet was what made them win the championship or look beautiful for the magazine cover. These examples appeal to your emotional need to believe the diet will produce the results you desperately crave. This social proof further sponsors the theory while also emotionally motivating you to adopt the diet.

Both the scientific evidence and the social proof further reinforce this idea that eating right is incredibly important. Not only does it matter in a general sense, but now the scientific and social evidence proves that not only should you follow the diet, but you *need* to follow it. If you want to be a hero for the team you need to eat right. If you want to be sexy and attractive, you need to follow the rules. Examples like this bring you right back to the starting belief that eating right is important, not just in a general sense, but now it's important for you on an emotional level, and the whole cycle starts again with even more momentum.

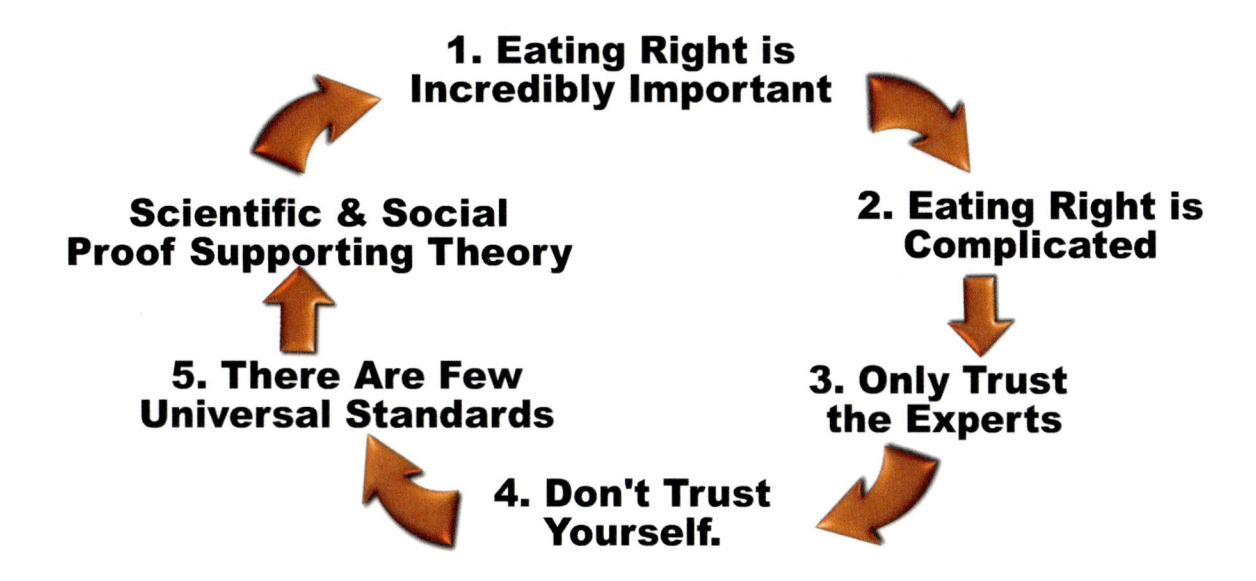

1. Eating Right is Incredibly Important
2. Eating Right is Complicated
3. Only Trust the Experts
4. Don't Trust Yourself.
5. There Are Few Universal Standards
Scientific & Social Proof Supporting Theory

The Eat Right Cycle produces dietary dogma that prevents real healthy eating.

Why I refuse to "eat right."

This cycle creates an eating philosophy I call "eating right." The very term of eating right implies that you are feeding yourself in a correct way according to a set of dogmatic rules someone invented. It's about staying on the straight and narrow while fighting yourself in an attempt to do the right thing. I highly take exception to this idea of eating right. It restricts your choices and options; it makes you your worst enemy and most of all it can even prevent you from fulfilling the cause of healthy eating in the first place.

Ending the Eat Right Cycle with the cause of healthy eating

The cause of healthy eating is simple. Its primary goal is the satisfaction and fulfillment of your needs through food. To put it simply, you have various needs and appetites and the entire reason to eat something, anything at all, is to satisfy those needs.

I find the best way to describe healthy eating is to use the analogy of filling up a bucket. You have a calorie bucket, a protein bucket, a vitamin C bucket and so on. Even things like eating for pleasure or social enjoyment have their bucket. Each bucket represents a single appetite or need that you must fill to be happy and healthy. Your mission is to fill as many of your "buckets" as possible without causing any of them to run empty or make them overflow.

If you can manage to fill your appetites optimally without overflow, you'll have all of the benefits of a healthy diet without any negative consequences. Everything you eat will serve a helpful purpose in supporting both your body and mind.

Appetite Buckets

Unsatisfied   Over-Full   Satisfied

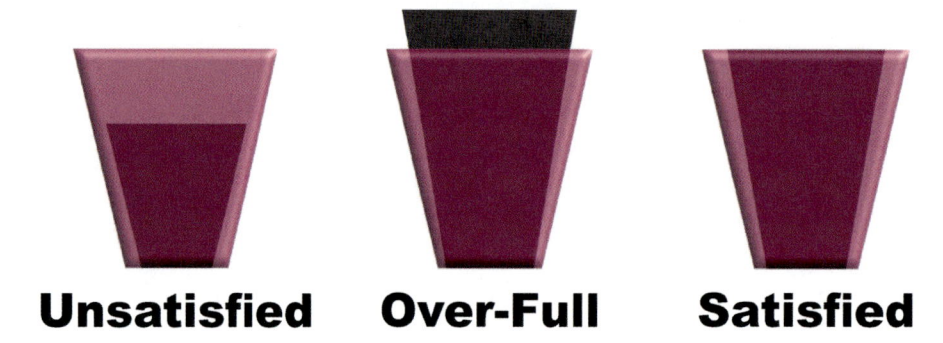

The goal of healthy eating is to hit that "Goldilocks zone" where everything is just right.

The challenge with achieving fulfillment is that everyone has different size appetite buckets to satisfy. One person may have a much bigger calorie bucket than another person so eating 3,000 will optimally fill up their bucket while the same amount of calories might cause the other person's bucket to overflow. Even though the number of calories is the same, it may be healthy for one person but not as healthy for someone else. You might require more fiber than your friend, or you may not need as much calcium as someone else. No general dietary recommendation will optimally satisfy everyone's appetites. All of the guidelines about how much you should eat are general guidelines. They are a base number to start with and then you make adjustments according to your needs.

In addition to having your unique needs, your appetites can change due to any number of lifestyle influences. You may have needed 4,000 calories when playing sports back in college, but now you have a desk job, and your calorie bucket has shrunk down to 2,600. Maybe you were fine with cereal for breakfast in the past, but now that you're starting a new weight lifting routine you find you need some more protein to keep from feeling famished by mid-morning.

Healthy eating vs. eating right

The phrases healthy eating and eating right may hold the same meaning for many people, but I believe they couldn't be more different. The first big difference is eating right and healthy eating is about satisfying separate objectives. While healthy eating is about fulfilling you and your needs, eating right is about satisfying the rules of a dogma. Healthy eating helps you achieve optimal health and fitness by learning about what is best for you personally and then applying those lessons while making adjustments as you go along. Eating right is based on the theory that there is an optimal way for you to eat, regardless of personal differences, and the best way to achieve optimal health is to shoehorn yourself within the rules of the program.

The next big difference is that when it comes to eating right, your desires and appetites are something you need to resist. You need to toughen up and stay disciplined while using willpower to follow the rules whether you like it or not. All of the cravings, hunger or unsatisfied desires are proof that you're fighting the good fight.

Since healthy eating is about satisfaction, things like cravings, guilt, constant hunger and unfulfilled appetites are signs that the diet is *not* healthy. The very act of eating is done to *remove* stress from your life rather than cause it. Stress is not the sign of a healthy diet. It's the sign of a poor diet and the more stress you experience, the less healthy your diet is.

Lastly, the biggest difference between healthy eating and eating right is their general approach to how you should change your diet to improve yourself. Most of the theories about eating right focus on what you need to remove from the menu, be it meat, dairy, fat, sugar or grains. These methods come from the observation that many people's buckets are overflowing due to popular dietary trends. The plan with eating right is to restrict certain foods to prevent those buckets from over filling. Meanwhile, other foods are encouraged with little restraint. It's this eat-this don't-eat-that idea that certain foods are always bad for you, and other foods are always right for you.

Healthy eating does not use this black and white approach. The goal is never to empty certain overflowing buckets but to satisfy all of your appetites. Instead of taking things out and restricting your choices healthy eating places all options on the table. Nothing is off limits with the possible exception of foods that trigger allergies and sensitivities. When satisfying your various appetites is the goal, your relationship to food changes in a big way. Now there is no dividing line between what foods are good or bad. You're no longer encouraged to eat as little of one thing, and as much of another. Now any food that can bring you satisfaction and fulfillment is healthy regardless of what it is. If you eat it, and it removes some stress, or supports your body, then it's good for you. On the other hand, any food that does not satisfy your needs, or causes stress, is not very healthy.

Eating Right	**Healthy Eating**
- Remove Bad Foods	- All Foods Are Available
- Always Eat Good Foods	- Aim to Satisfy Your Needs
- Fight Cravings & Desires	- Keep a Flexible Diet
- Don't Trust Yourself	- Listen to your Body and Mind

This perspective makes food selection more of a massive gray area rather than a black or white scenario. While it may not make healthy eating as simple as "eat this don't eat that" it does give you both the freedom to eat however you wish while simultaneously giving you the potential to fulfill your needs optimally.

There is no such thing as a healthy or unhealthy food

Another way the healthy eating approach turns eating right on its head is the way it looks at the potential health benefits of food. When it comes to eating right, certain foods are forever on the healthy or unhealthy side of the division line. With healthy eating, that division line can move at any time. Foods that are often considered healthy may not be the best choice while foods that are often considered unhealthy may potentially bring benefit and therefore be healthy.

Believing a particular food is always healthy or unhealthy is like a mechanic assuming a particular tool is always best regardless of what the job requires. While there are generalizations about what is healthy or not, it's important to allow flexibility in your diet. The only way you can manage your ever-changing appetites is to adopt a flexible approach to eating.

The biggest threat to your healthy eating is fear

Eating right is often based on fear and avoidance. The theory is that if you avoid all of the bad foods you'll have the fit, healthy and sexy body you want. Just open up any diet book and you'll find entire chapters of scientific and social proof convincing you that eating certain things is just straight up bad, wrong and maybe even a little bit immoral. This perspective creates the artificial rules of eating right by scaring you with the threat that bad things happen if you eat the wrong foods. At the same time, it promises you'll stay safe, lean, confident and sexy as long as you stick to those rules.

I used to believe this for a long time, but eventually, I came to understand that success in fitness, and life, doesn't come from always playing it safe and avoiding bad things. Sure, you don't want to be reckless, but no one ever made their dreams come true by avoiding mistakes. Despite this, the fear instilled by eating right can be just as unhealthy as the foods the diet claims to be bad. It doesn't matter what the latest research says about High Fructose Corn Syrup or the antibiotics used in meat production. All of that stuff is downright super food compared to the fear you ingest through eating right dogmas. Fear holds your potential in check while keeping a constant level of stress over your head. Let me give you an example of just how potent and dangerous fear can be from one of my history classes.

I once had a class in college where we studied military propaganda from the Second World War. We looked at posters, listened to radio broadcasts and even watched TV commercials containing both American and Japanese propaganda. At the heart of all of these materials was a driving message that the citizens of one country should fear and despise the citizens of another. It was often disguised as a " service bulletin" or a public health announcement, but in truth, it was a national message telling people to hate and fear other people.

Some years later I took on a project where I began reading a bunch of fad diet and fat loss books just to "keep up with the times." I hadn't even read more than a few pages before I felt like I was back in that college class reading materials convincing me that there was an evil empire I should despise, fear and fight. Only this time the propaganda wasn't against the people of another country but rather certain foods or ingredients.

After reading a few of the books, I started to feel my attitude towards food change. Whereas before, food was a good part of my life, I started looking at it as the enemy. I felt a dark cloud overshadow every food choice I made, and that cloud even darkened the times between meals. My mood was profoundly influenced by what I did or didn't eat, and I started to stress about what I was potentially going to eat in the future. Everything felt like it was in a downward spiral. It was a struggle with my appetites and desires. It was a fight with other people I was eating with too. It was even a struggle just to figure out what to order on a menu. However, despite all of this stress, I also became infatuated with the feeling of control.

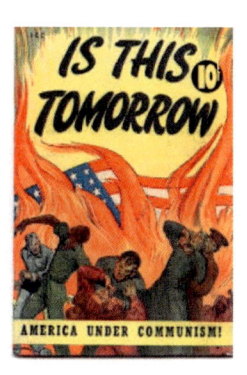

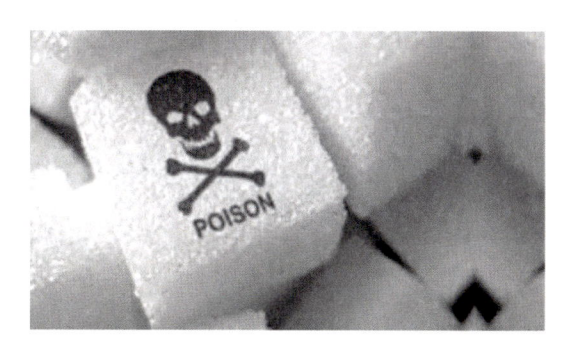

On the left a poster from the Vietnam War era. The right is an image promoting low sugar diets. All propaganda serves the same purpose which is to keep you fearful and obedient.

The most dangerous thing about fear is it gives you the illusion of power and control. When people fear something they feel in control when they take action against that it. During war, fear gives the fighter the sense of power as they fight against their enemy. When it comes to fitness, fear gives you the false impression that you can control your body, and even your life if you can just manage to eat right. Every time you abide by the rules of the diet you feel secure knowing you are vanquishing the oppressive powers that hold you down.

The only problem is this feeling of control is a complete illusion. Fear makes you seek security by building walls around yourself which end up becoming your personal prison. You feel safe from threats, but you're also limiting your freedom. The more the fear seeps into your mind, the thicker and higher you build those walls. It's just like when kids refuse to get out of bed in fear of the monster under their bed. Even though they want a drink or need to use the bathroom, their fear makes them feel secure as long as they stay in bed.

One of the most convincing tools of propaganda is "science." Scientific fact is often used to add credibility to the latest propaganda. Hitler used science to justify his atrocities. So did the Japanese and even the Americans. It doesn't matter if it's not right or bent more ways than a pretzel, people are nervous during times of uncertainty such as war or when they are unhappy with the state of their body. This change can make anyone vulnerable to whatever answers come around promising an end to that uncertainty through control and power. As history has proven, human beings will resort to crimes against humanity if it means taking control of a scary or uncertain situation. If fear can motivate people to kill each other, it can most certainly make people adopt dietary rules that jeopardize their potential to eat healthily.

Tackling the fear of the self

It's bad enough the dietary propaganda tells you to fear certain foods, but it even tells you to worry about yourself. Many experts claim that you're an addicted out of control person, and you need the confining walls of eating right to save you from yourself. Once again, the message promising security through fear rings clear. If you can just manage to eat right according to their rules, you will break the addictions and primal desires responsible for your downfall.

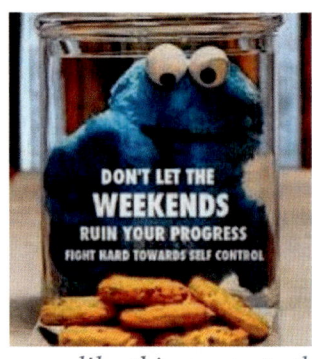

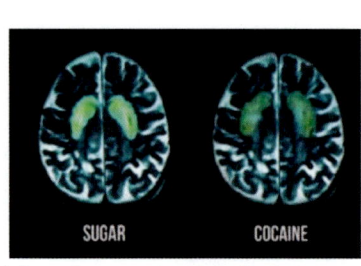

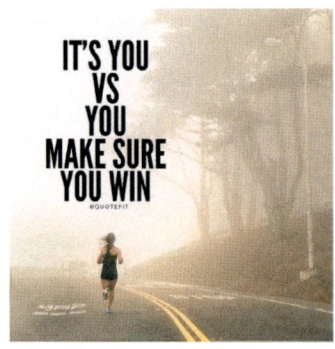

Messages like this promote the idea that eating right is supposed to be a struggle against your desires and appetites.

With healthy eating, there is nothing to fear and nothing to avoid. There's nothing to fight against or do battle with on a daily basis. Not carbohydrates. Not sugar or meat and most certainly not yourself. You may be asking me "You mean to tell me I have permission to eat anything and everything without any restrictions at all?! I don't have to fight myself, so that means if I want to eat 5 pints of ice cream I just let myself indulge? It sounds like you're suggesting dietary suicide." I know exactly how you feel. After all, that's the whole story behind eating right that creates all of that fear. It's the story that tells you you'll fall into an endless pit of severe consequences if you don't hold fast to the rules of eating right. Free fall is inevitable and your need the diet to save you from yourself and all of the evil out there.

The solution to the fearful motivations of eating right

As I mentioned earlier, success doesn't come from avoiding adverse consequences. After all, a bike racer doesn't win just because they don't get lost and avoid crashing. You don't get a 5-star review simply by showing up to work on time. You don't receive the spoils of healthy eating by avoiding the evil. You gain the rewards by seeking beneficial outcomes!

The biggest problem with eating right is it sets incredibly low standards. When a diet focuses on avoiding certain foods, the rule is simple, yet it leaves plenty of opportunities to still fall short. One of the biggest examples of this was back when eating right meant keeping to a low-fat diet. This simple rule left the door wide open for all sorts of unhealthy eating. People avoided fatty cuts of meat, eggs, and even some types of fish.

At the same time, the simple rule of eating low fat meant that low-fat cookies, cakes, and candy were perfectly healthy. Following the simple rule of eating low fat caused many to over eat some foods and under eat others. As a result, some appetites remained chronically unmet while others are overfed. Eating a bunch of fat-free cookies while avoiding a plate of eggs might seem unhealthy today, but back then it was perfectly acceptable. Eating right only meant keeping to the low standard of eating as little fat as possible.

These days, many modern theories on how to eat right criticize the old notion of the low-fat diet. The new theories claim that low-fat eating was a misleading way to eat right, but now the experts have it all figured out. This time, they've got it right with the latest theory stating that eating right is about avoiding carbs, or sugar, or meat or whatever. It feels great to be living in this enlightened age where science has finally unlocked the secret to eating right. However, the veterans of fitness see the latest fads as just the latest turn in the never ending cycle. As the line dividing good foods from bad food shifts, various appetites become overfed while others remain chronically deprived. This imbalance fuels the next round of dietary dogmas based on which foods people eat in excess, and what other foods they don't eat enough. The latest dogmatic fads become popular and our fitness culture falls down yet another rabbit hole.

The four appetites of healthy eating

When I claim that eating right sets, a low standard I mean it. You can have the cleanest diet and be 100% free of the latest dietary demons yet still fall drastically short of a truly healthy diet. You cannot eat healthy through just adhering to just one or two trendy rules. Instead, healthy eating aims to fulfill four basic appetites that are as primal as life itself. Through trying to satisfy each of these appetites, your diet will naturally balance itself out and provide you with the best chance of gaining all of the benefits that can come from healthy eating. If your dietary standards are only about nutrition or eating something that tastes good, you neglect the other appetites which can still bring you stress. Since the healthiness of a diet is about removing stress from your life, any eat-right dogma that fails to satisfy one of these appetites is still inadequate.

Appetite #1 Physical hunger

Hunger is one of the most primal motivations people ever experience. If your hunger is intense enough, it can override your desire for any other appetite including sleep and sex. Hunger can cloud your thinking, significantly decrease your physical performance and make your willpower fall apart like a sand castle in a hurricane. Taking care of your hunger is one of the healthiest and most powerful things you can do for yourself. Once you get your hunger under control the floodgates of potential open up.

It's for this reason that a healthy diet *must* satisfy your hunger. It sounds simple enough, but the notion of eating right has done a lot of damage over the years towards allowing you to satisfy your hunger.

The first reason is that whole idea that you shouldn't trust yourself, and you need to fight your desires to eat right. Much of the time this means fighting against or ignoring your hunger. People train themselves to eat according to the rules of the diet which sometimes means both abstaining from food when they are hungry as well as forcing themselves to eat when they are not. They learn that hunger is something to fight against which ends up being a fight against their self.

They see their hunger as an uncontrolled demon they must wrestle into submission or else they will lose themselves to it.

These ideas come from the notion that the human body will constantly ask for food and that people will eat whenever they can. Therefore, the diet is offered as a form of salvation to save the person from themselves. The irony is it's the very rules of the dogma that are creating the endless desire for food and long stretches of hunger. After all, the hunger for food is just like any other appetite. Once it's fulfilled the hunger goes away, and it's no longer an issue.

Unfortunately, many dogmatic approaches to food can cause swings between deprivation and over indulgence. When someone refuses to give into their hunger they build up a lot of both physical and mental stress that can only be satisfied with food. Naturally, the satisfaction from finally eating removes the stress of hunger very quickly, but it rarely stops there as you continue to eat until they are overfed. These binges can make you feel out of control and support the idea that you will eat in self-destructive ways. When your hunger is satisfied the stress is gone and with it may be a sense of guilt or regret over eating so much. In this state, it can be tempting to "get back on track" and resolve to stick with the diet with more willpower vowing to fight harder, and the whole cycle begins anew.

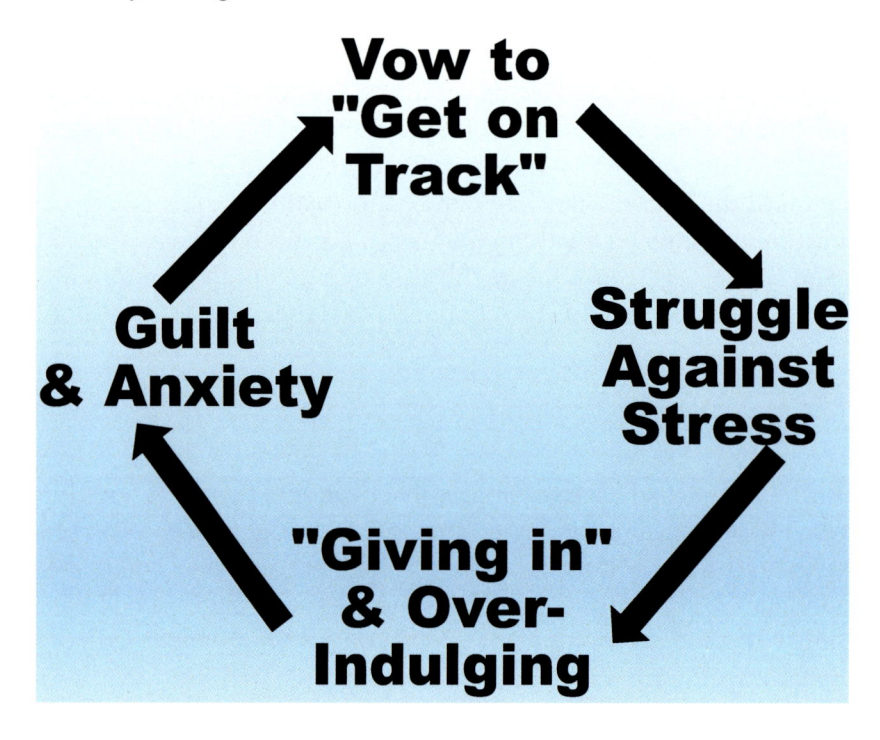

The cycle of hunger and deprivation can create an endless cycle that makes you feel helpless and out of control.

The issue with the hunger cycle is that both fighting hunger and giving into it can cause you to feel like you're out of control. It creates feelings of vulnerability and damages self-esteem with each revolution.

Healthy eating avoids these swings between massive hunger and over eating. When your goal is to eat for satisfaction, you learn to avoid both of these excessive states. You eat when you're hungry to create a state of comfort. You also stop eating when you have reached a point of satisfaction but are not overfed. By avoiding both extreme hunger and overfeeding you're much more in control, and you don't have the adverse effects of either.

Appetite #2 Pleasure and enjoyment

Just like hunger, the joy, and pleasure you gain from food is also something eating right theories claim you need to fight. Supposedly, if something tastes great, it's because that food probably contains something that's unhealthy. A lot of people point to the idea that humans have a natural desire for sweet foods. It's also a common idea that various food companies have "engineered" their foods to be sweet, fatty and salty in such a way to make people addicted. I've even heard some people say that if the food tastes superb, then it shouldn't be eaten! So according to these theories, eating right means avoiding pleasure from food.

All of these ideas made sense to me back when I was trying to eat right, but now I think they are absolute insanity. Just as with hunger, the desire for pleasure is one of the most important aspects of a healthy diet. Forcing yourself to avoid the pleasures of food is just as bad as avoiding food itself.

Food is more than fuel

Many theories on eating right attempt to downgrade food as nothing more than mere fuel for the body. The idea is that if you eat primarily for the sake of meeting your nutritional needs, then you won't overeat, you won't eat junk food, and you will be healthy as a horse. This idea also comes with the notion that your desire to eat for pleasure and enjoyment are inner demons you need to resist. Going out and having a few beers with friends or enjoying dessert after dinner are seen as sinful and unhealthy extravagant choices that lead to an expanding waistline and disease. I used to hold to these ideas myself, but now I see them for the ancient archaic approach they are.

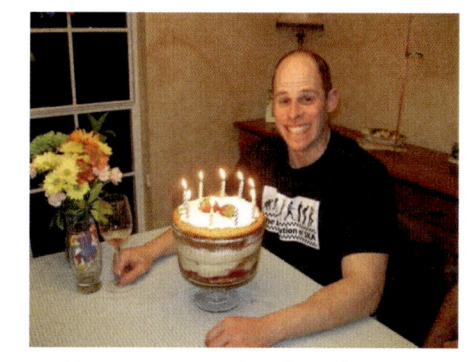

Food can be, and should be an enjoyable part of your life. The scent, taste, and texture of foods are what poets write stanzas about, and songwriters write about. Jimmy Buffett didn't sing about a Cheeseburger in Paradise because he needed an optimal protein to carbohydrate ratio after a workout.

Nothing tastes as good as skinny feels, except for my Mom's Strawberry truffle.

It's more than just the physical pleasure that comes from food. Eating also brings social enjoyment as well. I couldn't imagine a holiday season without my Mom's Christmas cookies and who ever thought of hosting a super bowl party with nothing but bottled water and raw kale chips? Withholding pleasure indefinitely is not the way to a healthy diet. I'm not saying you should give in to every whim and small appetite that comes your way, but to try and degrade food as nothing more than a means to convey nutrition is simply unnecessary at best and stressful at worst.

Appetite #3 Energy

Your diet is a massive influence towards your energy level. If your diet is not very healthy, your blood sugar and nutritional support will be all over the place sending you through peaks of high energy followed by deep lows of sluggish fatigue.

Mental stress can also drain your energy. A healthy diet shouldn't require a lot of mental effort to maintain. The more work your mind and emotions have to do to feed yourself the less energy, there is left over for the other important tasks in your life. This is why one of the biggest goals of healthy eating is to maintain a high energy level throughout the day. Eating should leave you feeling awake and refreshed not sluggish and sleepy.

Appetite #4 Nutrition and physical support

Lastly, we couldn't discuss healthy eating without addressing the importance of quality nutrition. The human body is incredibly robust and can survive with very limited nutritional resources. That said, the more restrictive your diet is, the more stress your body has to face to operate with the scarce resources. The more nutrients you can potentially consume the less stress your diet will create.

The healthy eating net

The great thing about these four appetites is they all support each other while also keeping themselves in check. For example, the appetite of hunger will help ensure you eat enough to satisfy your need for energy while maintaining your consumption in check. Both eating too much and eating too little will compromise your energy level. The appetite for pleasure will help prevent you from feeling deprived and restricted, plus it will also keep your consumption in check. Hunger increases the pleasure from food, but there is a diminishing rate of return as you continue eating. Have you ever noticed how the first bite of something is the best, but after a while the taste and sensation of eating that same food decreases? It can even become a personal challenge to finish a meal or to clean your plate because the positive sensations of eating diminished so much they became negative.

And then we have the drive for better nutrition. The more nutrients a food or meal has, the more potential pleasure there is from eating it. Including a wide variety of natural ingredients improves the taste and texture of a meal as opposed to a meal of just one or two bland processed ingredients. Lastly, bringing more nutritional resources to a meal contributes to support the chemical reactions that improve energy and heighten awareness.

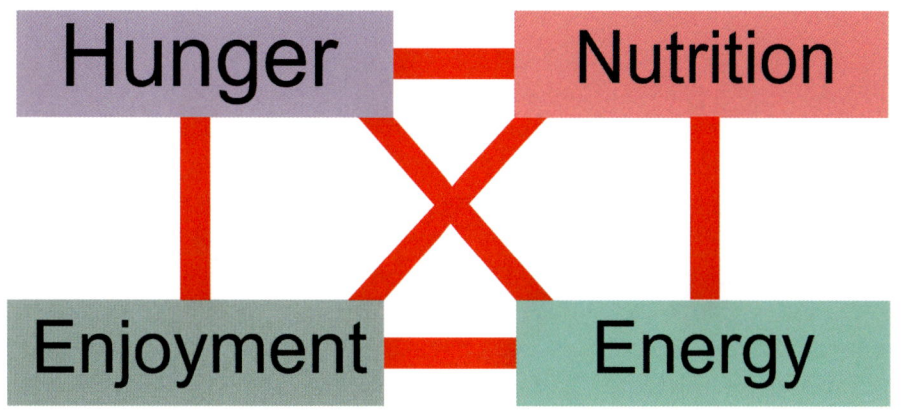

Each of the 4 appetites is an influence towards the other 3. This promotes a healthy diet by ensuring the satisfaction of each appetite while also keeping each desire in check.

Essential Tips for healthy eating

Just like all root causes, how you fulfill the cause of healthy eating is unique to you, and your methods will change with time. Even so, here are a few core principles I recommend to make healthy eating easier, simpler and much more rewarding for the long term.

1. **Listen and trust yourself**

Your body is the best diet advisor in the world. With every bite, your body is sending you signals about how it feels regarding how beneficial that food is. Listen to it, and try to understand what it's telling you.

2. **Maintain consistency in your diet**

Keeping a consistent diet will do wonders for both body and mind. Just like with exercise, your body will adapt to how you feed it. The more consistency you have in your diet, the easier it is to keep both your body and mind happy. Your body will know what's coming and be ready for it. You'll also sync your appetite with meal times to help you avoid getting caught with bouts of hunger. Consistency also makes it much easier to improve your diet and make it healthier.

3. **Use a wide variety of foods**

The best way to boost both the enjoyment, as well as the nutritional profile of a meal, is to include a broad range of foods. Compare a salad with nine different ingredients over a simple slice of ham and cheese between two slices of bread. Which do you think will taste better? Which do you think will fill you up and satisfy your palate? The greater variety of foods will be sure to improve both the enjoyment of the food, plus the nutritional value.

4. **Control your food environment**

Your dietary environment consists of the food choices you have around you. Examples can include the food in your home and works environment. Don't forget to consider food options like a vending machine down the hall or the coffee shop you pass on your way to the bus stop.

While there are influences in your environment you have little control over, like a coffee shop next to your office, managing the forces you can control will go a long way towards controlling your diet. If you have healthier choices readily at hand, it will be easier to make healthier decisions. I use something I like to call the stop light strategy. It's very simple as you self-categorize foods into green, yellow, and red light foods.

Green light foods are healthy choices you want to eat every day. These foods are the ones you want to make sure you keep readily available in your immediate environment such as your home and at work. Examples might include a bag of almonds in your desk drawer for when you get a snack craving or a bowl of fruit on the kitchen counter at home.

Yellow light foods are foods you eat in moderation or very sparingly and you don't have trouble doing so. If you enjoy a handful of potato chips now and then, you might keep a bag in the back of a cupboard. This way, you have access to your occasional treats and indulgences, but they're not always tempting you every time you walk into the kitchen or open up the refrigerator.

Red light foods are foods you have a hard time eating in moderation. If you struggle to keep yourself from eating a full pint of Ben & Jerry's, it's a good idea to keep ice cream out of your home and work environment. Keeping red light food out of your environment doesn't mean you have to eliminate ice cream from your diet. You can still enjoy it; you just make a special trip to get an ice cream cone. By making it slightly harder to indulge in your favorite treats, you automatically make it easier to satisfy less of them and greatly decrease your chances of overeating.

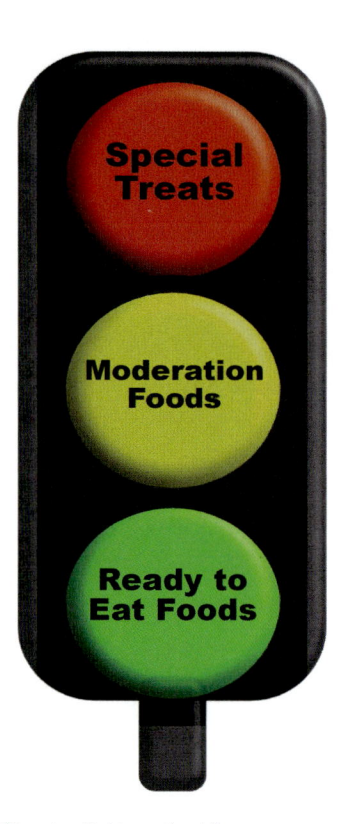

The stoplight method for controlling your food environment.

Keep in mind; foods may shift around within your personal stop light system. Yellow light foods may become red light foods and vice versa. Keep in mind that it's important, to be honest with yourself about how well you can control the consumption of the foods within your environment.

5. **Prepare your food**

For all the debate and confusion over diet out there, eating well boils down to three factors; what you eat, how much you eat, and when you eat. Preparing your food goes a very long way in helping you master all three of those components.

Consider the difference between making your lunch versus being at the mercy of whatever is available in the cafeteria. When you make your food, you can pack whatever you like and leave out whatever you don't. If you make yourself a bowl of hot food or a sandwich you're in control of exactly what goes into it and how much of each ingredient you include. Making your food also means you can have your food readily available in your dietary environment so if you want a snack, you have easy access to it.

Compare this with always going to the cafeteria or a food shop during a designated lunch break. When you get your food prepared by someone else you have far less control over what you have available. If someone else is making you a sandwich they may put more cheese or oil on it, then you may have put on yourself. Plus, the portion size may be much bigger than what you need. You also don't have the freedom to get that food whenever you want. If hunger hits like a wrecking ball before a mid-morning meeting, you don't have the luxury to grab something quick to satisfy you through the meeting.

You don't have to be a five-star chef to make your food. In fact, you can probably make much better food than what you would get at most restaurants with a little creativity and practice.

I recommend starting off by making a list of some of your favorite dishes you eat at restaurants. Once you have that list, do a search online for some of the "best" recipes for those foods. If you're a big fan of the spaghetti at your local Italian restaurant, see if you can find a way to make a similar dish or maybe even a better one. Perhaps you'd prefer ground sausage to ground beef in the sauce, or maybe you like things on the spicy side. Whatever makes your mouth water, turn your attention towards making better versions of the foods you enjoy.

Another tip is to make your food in bulk. I fully understand that cooking and preparing meals can be a chore, especially at the end of a long work day. When you make your foods in bulk, you can store them in ready-to-eat containers for a quick grab on the go meal. That way you have something healthier, easier and more satisfying right in your kitchen as opposed to having to order take out.

One of the biggest reasons to prepare your food is the efficiency it can bring to your day. Just think how easy it is to walk into your kitchen and grab something to eat. In contrast, you can get in your car, drive to a restaurant, wait for a table, wait for a menu, wait to place your order, wait for your food, wait for them to bring back your check and then drive home.

The value of finite appetites

Sometimes people don't quite believe that fulfillment is a good goal to have when it comes to healthy eating. Due to years of trying to eat right, they feel they have appetites that are never satisfied and seeking to fulfillment would mean eating loads of junk food every day. Some folks have told me they could eat ice cream or chocolate forever and never get tired of it. I once felt this way myself. I even had days when I would eat 2 or 3 pints of Ben & Jerry's ice cream without feeling like I would ever get my fill. This feeling of a never ending appetite can come from many sources. The first reason is that many theories on eating right are based on the idea that it's healthy to keep particular appetites unfed as much as possible. Those appetites as always unfulfilled so you never feel like you can get enough.

Another reason for an endless desire to eat is when an appetite or desire is unmet because eating doesn't address the particular source of stress you're experiencing. An example might be if you're stressing over a project at work and you attempt to alleviate that stress by overeating sweets. While the sweets may bring you some pleasure in the short term, they do little to reduce the actual stress from work. Since the sweets do little to relieve the stress, you remain unsatisfied no matter how much you eat. Always remember, satisfying an appetite is both easy and efficient when you give yourself exactly what you want. If you refuse to "give in" you'll consume loads of resources trying to become satisfied through other means.

Lastly, there is always the possibility of a physical imbalance like a hormone level that's off a bit which can cause you to feel constantly hungry. If this is the case, you'll need to get tested by your doctor and seek medical help to balance things back out

Regardless of the reason, the cause of the endless appetite is the same. You have a desire or need for something, and you're not fulfilling that desire. If you're lonely, you can eat cookies all day long, but it won't do anything to alleviate your appetite for companionship. If you're never allowing yourself to eat enough carbs, you'll always have an unfulfilled desire to eat carbohydrates no matter how much spaghetti squash you eat. If you have a hormonal imbalance, then your brain can't quite tell when you've had enough. In all cases, obtaining satisfaction of your appetite is the solution. Nothing cures hunger and desire like fulfilling that desire. Avoiding "giving in" and satisfying that desire is will ensure you always suffer from it.

It might be hard to imagine, but all appetites are very finite. When you give yourself exactly what you want, the desire for that thing ceases to exist. The key is understanding what your appetites are and then fulfilling them as efficiently as possible without playing games with yourself. Your appetites are always on a diminishing rate of return when you satisfy yourself. Have you ever started indulging in a treat and the first few bites feel like heaven, but somewhere along the way you were eating just to clean your plate? This is an example of how your appetites are finite. Also, the more you overeat, the most stressful eating becomes. Your body is not built to eat massive quantities after you've had enough.

Above all, healthy eating is as much an art as it is a science. It's a balance between your resources and appetites to create an environment that helps remove stress from your life rather than cause it. I know this chapter may bring up more questions than answer and for now, that's what I wanted to do by writing it. While eating right helps you feel secure and attempts to remove uncertainty about how to eat, healthy eating can cause you to feel like you're not quite sure about what how you should eat. I know this risk might feel a little uneasy, but I promise you it's a good thing. It's this very uncertainty that will fuel the ultimate appetite of all, which is the desire always to learn how to eat better which is at the heart of learning the skill of healthy eating.

8: The Delta Principles

Fitness Independence is about distilling fitness down to the essential rules you need to achieve success. Through refining and simplifying the rules of fitness you can spend less, gain more and experience a much greater degree of flexibility within your lifestyle.

Up until now, I've been focusing on the root causes, the very essence of what it takes to reach the most popular fitness goals within our fitness culture. With what I've covered so far, you're already miles ahead of most people when it comes to getting in shape. Even so, understanding the cause of your goal is only a portion of what you need to understand. There are still more principles to cover, principles that can make or break your success regardless of how well you understand the cause of your goal. These are what I call the Delta Principles. Just like the 3 legs of a tripod, each one is essential. Leave just one of these principles out and you stand no chance of success. However, if you have all of these in your program you cannot fail. The more you fulfill all 5 of these principles, the more success you enjoy, guaranteed. There's a lot at stake here so let's not waste time and get right to it, shall we?

Delta principle #1 Consistency

First, we have one of the most essential fitness principles of all, consistency. No matter what your goals are or what makes you unique, consistent habits are the backbone to your success. Building a great body is just like constructing a massive structure brick by brick. Each meal, exercise, and workout you do is just like a single brick. Eating well for a day or giving 100% effort to your workout might feel like a lot of work, but those short term actions are only tiny contributions in the grand scheme of things. The only way those small influences can add up to a meaningful result is the power of repetition and nothing builds up repetition quickly like consistency.

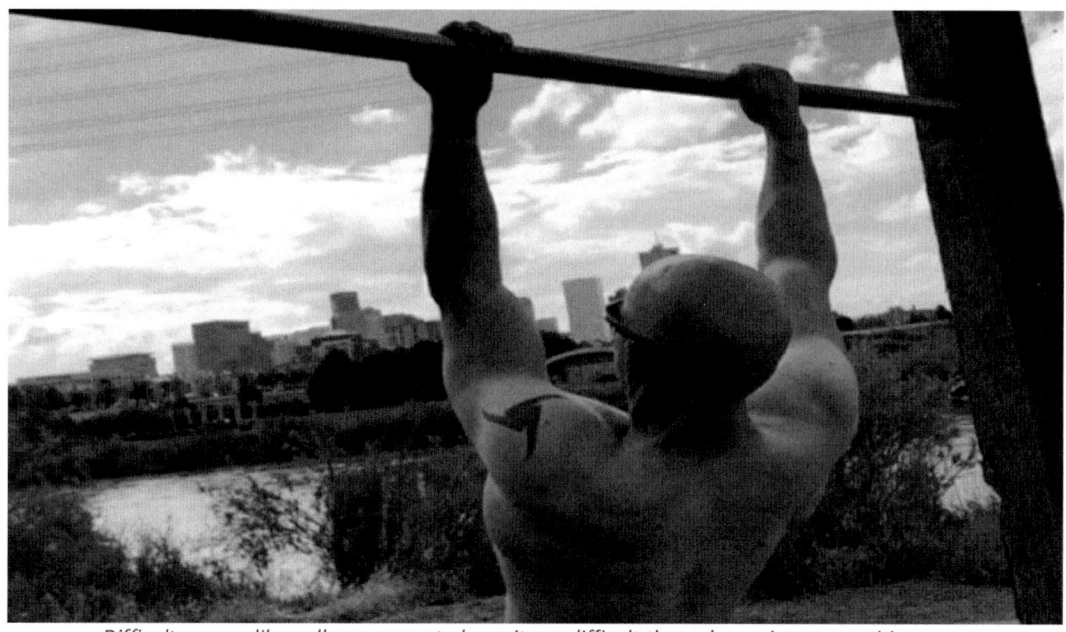

Difficult moves, like pull ups, cease to be quite so difficult through consistent repetition.

The power of repetition significantly increases your chances of success no matter how much the odds are against you when starting out. Repetition can also take power away from you as well. You could have every advantage in the world, but a lack of consistent repetition will leave you floundering against the winds of change. Consistency is why the long shots win and the heavily favored loose.

Don't worry about set and rep routines or protein to carbohydrate ratios just yet. All of that stuff doesn't mean a thing until you get your diet and exercise habits consistently established first. Consistent repetition is the foundation upon which all of your success builds upon.

Threats to your consistency

Keeping consistent habits may seem obvious, but several false ideals are floating around our fitness culture that suggest it's not important or even bad. One of the most notable theories is this idea that variety will stimulate change in the body. Some experts even claim you don't want to use a consistent diet or exercise routine in fear that your body will get used to it.

You can first see where these ideas jump the logic tracks by the words used to describe how you want to keep the body "confused" and to keep your muscles "guessing." If you want to condition your body towards any goal, confusion and guessing are the very last things you want.

Training your body is just like training and learning any other skill. It's much easier to grow and develop your abilities when the lessons are simple, clear, and repetitive. "Mixing it up" with a ton of variety and fluff causes your program to become fragmented and diluted. It makes even the most basic techniques a lot harder to learn not to mention much more expensive.

Another false idea is you need such inconsistency because you don't want your muscles or body to get used to the diet or workout routine. Supposedly, once your body gets used to the routine, then it stops changing and you hit a plateau. Again, this is absolute nonsense!

You *want* your body to get used to that routine. You *want* your muscles to get used to the training. You *want* your body to get used to the diet. Not only do you want to get used to your habits, but you want to get used to them as quickly as possible. When your body gets used to a routine you have accomplished what you wanted it to do; it adapted! You grew muscle. You developed coordination. Your body improved how it moves. If you struggle with an exercise, and then it feels like you've "gotten used to it" it means you've become more fit!

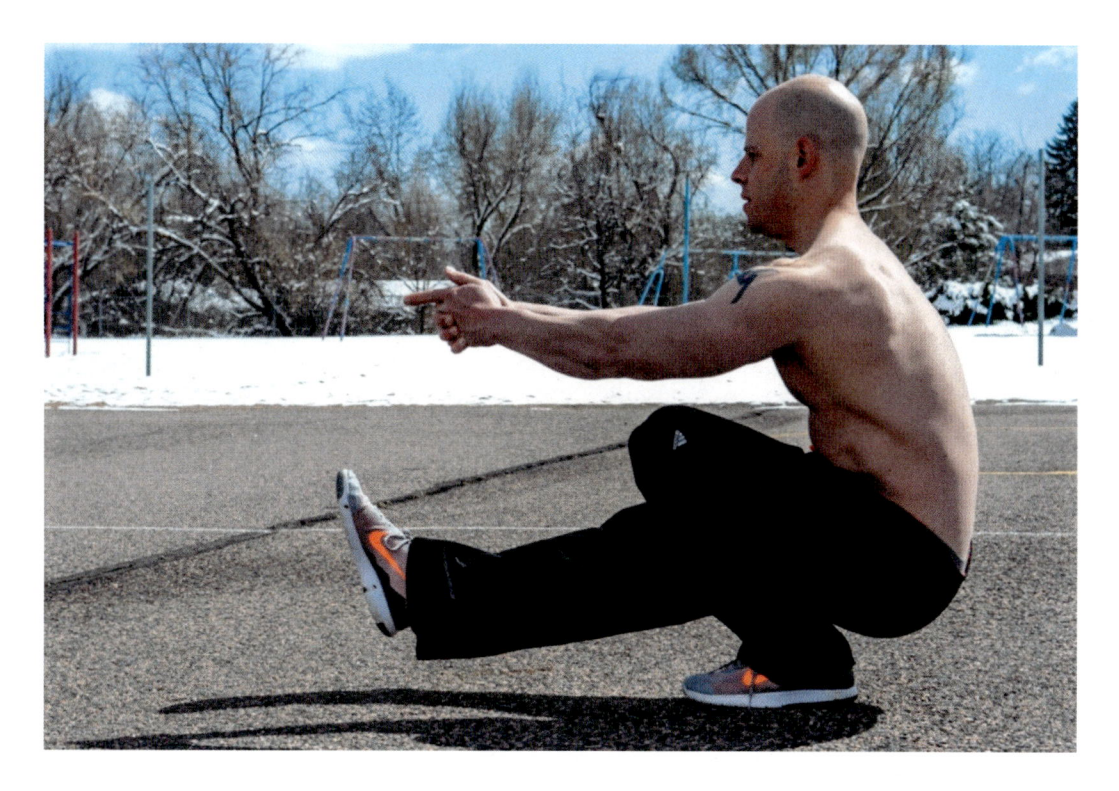

The only way to learn how to squat on one leg is to get used to squatting on two legs first.

The idea of muscle confusion and keeping the body guessing is akin to being lost. Sure you're always experiencing something new, as the scenery changes, but do you want to wander around while wasting your resources hoping you'll end up where you want to go? Of course not! You want the most direct route between where you are now and where you want to go and the best way to do that is to keep your habits simple, clear and consistent. However, don't mistake consistency with doing the exact same thing week after week. There is some change that needs to happen, and that change is the second Delta Principle of progression.

Delta principle #2 Progression

Having consistency doesn't mean you always do things the exact same way over and over again. While that sort of approach will help you maintain your progress, it will do almost nothing for achieving better results. You need to keep moving forward. You need to keep progressing.
If fitness could be sold by the bottle, you would find progression on the label under "active ingredients."

Progression is nothing short of magic. It packs your body full of muscle and strength. It sheds fat, erases the pain, and brings you more rewards for the same amount of effort. Also, don't forget that progression applies just as much to your diet as it does to exercise. Rather than "eating right" you always want to find little ways to progress your diet, so it becomes healthier and more fulfilling.
Progress is the answer to almost every diet and exercise question out there. It's just so darn unfortunate that so many people don't care too much about it. Hell, some people even

deliberately ignore it all together! Instead of seeking progression, they seek something else entirely; hard work.

Hard work vs. progression

Our fitness culture is obsessed with hard work. While hard work is usually a good thing, it can become costly and extremely unhealthy. The focus on hard work started with the "no pain no gain" mentality, and it's grown by leaps and bounds. People post on social media boasting about how hard their workout was or how much they are suffering from losing weight. It's become a worldwide contest over who can work the hardest and who can outwork the competition.
I fell under the hard work spell for years because I thought I would get results if I could just work hard enough.

I also fell for the simple idea that you get out of a program what you put into it. Believe me; there have been plenty of times when I've put a lot in but received very little in return.
It's true, you need to work very hard to achieve your goals, but relying on hard work alone is one of the biggest mistakes you can make in fitness. After all, hard work is nothing more than spending lifestyle resources. It's about spending time, money, energy and discipline. It's that whole promise that if you can spend enough then, you'll reach the promised land of six pack abs and blinding performance.

The hard work trap usually starts when you take your first few steps toward building a better body. You get off the couch and start doing squats while watching TV. You use a bit of discipline and order the grilled chicken salad in the cafeteria instead of pizza. You take a walk after work instead of downing a few beers. After a few weeks, you start to look and feel better, so you decide to crank things up a bit. Instead of walking 20 minutes you vow to walk for 40. You cut back on your afternoon snack of chocolate chip cookies and go for carrot sticks. You even spend some money on a doorway pull up bar. As the results come, you spend more resources and work harder. At this point, your mind has established a connection between working harder and getting results. You start believing you can achieve anything as long as you're willing to work hard enough for it.

This sort of situation sounds great, but it doesn't last forever. Lifestyle resources are finite which means you can only fulfill a few influences to a limited extent.

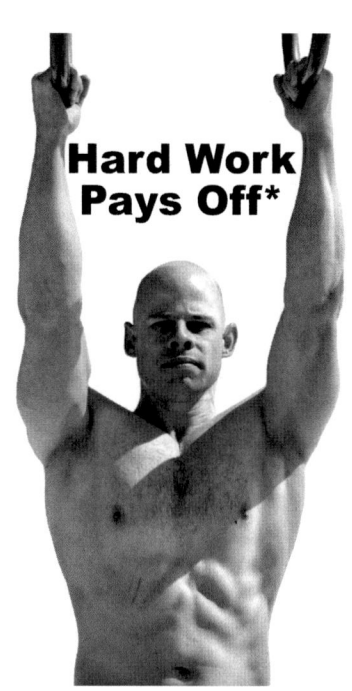

When combined with progression of skills and capabilities.

Eventually, you'll start to run empty, and your potential will quickly hit a dead end. Once you can't work any harder you hit the dreaded plateau where you're now busting your tail every day just to stay where you are. You lose hope of achieving your dream body and maybe even consider quitting. It may sound dreary, but this is your best possible outcome you can hope for from the work harder strategy.

If you don't submit to a plateau, you'll end up overworking which is when you overspend your lifestyle resources in the never ending pursuit of greater results. You spend more time working out instead of spending that time on other things like work, study or maintaining relationships. You can also spend the physical energy you simply don't have. Before too long, you're fighting nagging colds and aches and pains. Instead of leaping forward with the progress you're constantly recovering from one physical setback after another. Call it over training, overworking or overextending yourself, but the bottom line is you're spending lifestyle resources you are running low on. Your only two choices are to either stop moving forward or crash.

But wait! There is another option! Instead of banging your head against the wall to drive a square peg into a round hole, you can stop partaking in the fitness rat race and point yourself towards a horizon of potentially infinite rewards.

Achieving progression helps you break free of the diet and exercise rat race. It means you can keep moving forward without spending more resources. Your workouts can still take the same amount of time and energy yet you keep getting stronger. Your diet isn't any harder to stick to yet you look and feel better each week! Progression isn't about following some crazy formula or routine. It's learning and developing habits to further fulfill the cause of your goal. The more you accomplish the root causes, the better your results get, even if it doesn't cost you any additional time or energy. So instead of spending more time, money and energy and hoping for better results, you seek out ways to further fulfill the cause of your goal while keeping spending to a minimum.

A few more points about progression:

Progress comes in very small steps

One reason why so many people focus on hard work, instead of progression, is because hard work *feel*s more important. When you stagger out of the gym in a state of fatigue, it seems like you've done something monumental. When you use every ounce of self-control to avoid the cookie platter at a party, it feels like you've just made massive strides forward.

Progression doesn't always seem like a big deal. Most of the time, it doesn't come in a tidal wave of improvement but instead as a slow trickle. No one brags about having slightly more hamstring activation during their squats on Facebook. People don't boast at a party about how they are drinking only one beer instead of 4. It just doesn't seem sexy and newsworthy.

While super hard work might feel like you've just moved mountains if you haven't further fulfilled the cause of your goal you haven't made any headway. After all, treading water for 3 hours can be exhausting, but it won't get you any closer to dry land. Swimming in one direction for 5 minutes may not seem like much, but it does get you closer to your objective.

The Japanese have a great term for the progressive mindset called *Kaizen*. Kaizen means to make small daily improvements. It's a shame we don't have a term like that here in the west because taking small daily steps towards fulfilling your root causes will make the path to success very manageable and easier to sustain.

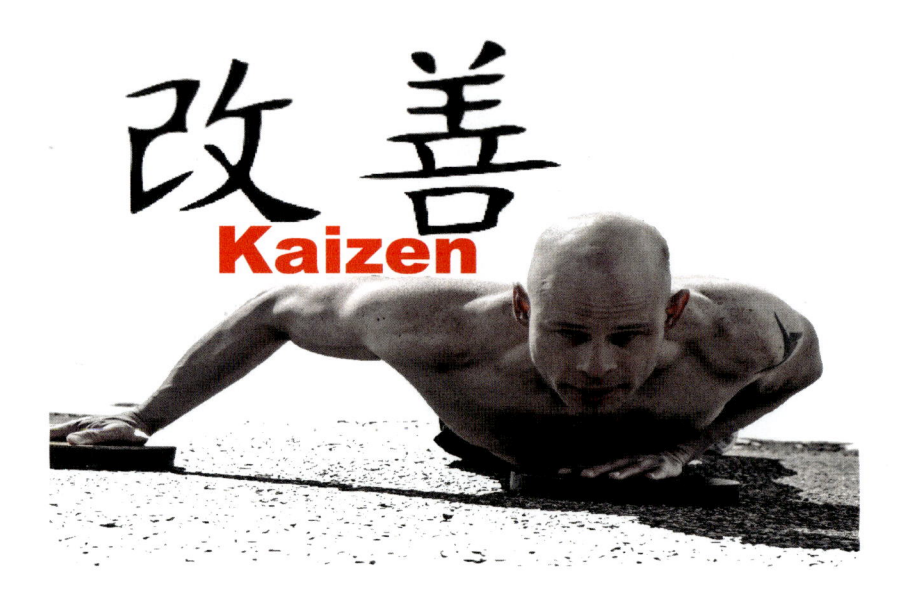

That's .05% more weight on my left arm from last time. I'm on my way!

I know you may be asking yourself "But Matt how will I know what steps to take to progress?" There are two answers to that question. The first is that understanding how to improve is part of the art and science of fitness. The path of progression is never fully known or understood. It's like walking through a fog where you can only see a few feet in front of you. All you can do is take the few steps you can see right in front of you. Then the next few feet will become apparent to you, and you can keep moving forward.

The second answer is much simpler. Just look for the next step you need to take and you will find it. If you are trying to lose weight, asking yourself how you can speed up your calorie expenditure or slow down your intake will make you more aware of what you should do. Once you are aware of the sort of actions you need to take to fulfill the cause of your goal you'll find opportunity every day to make a little progress.

This is why being aware of the cause of your goals is so key. It sharpens your awareness towards what influences your daily habits have towards that cause. If you keep an eye out for the opportunities to progress, they will become apparent.

Progression requires a target

I've always enjoyed games that involve aiming at a target. Be it archery, basketball or darts I've always become more proficient at hitting that target when I consistently practiced trying to hit it.

Can you imagine what would happen if you just randomly threw a basketball into the air, or threw darts into a wall? Even though you could spend the same amount of time and energy (still working hard), your capabilities wouldn't improve at all. Having a clear target to aim at with every repetition is the key to your progress. This is why you always need a goal in mind for every action you take. What is your target with the next set of pushups? Are you trying to do 20 reps? Are you trying to keep your elbows in tight? Are you aiming to touch the floor with every rep? What about with your diet? Are you seeking to include some protein at each meal? Maybe you're looking to stop eating before you feel stuffed. It doesn't matter what your target is just as long as you can further fulfill the cause of your goal by hitting it or at least come closer to hitting it.

Progression = happiness?

Over the years I've been privileged to witness a lot of people who become ecstatic over the progress they've made towards their goals. Every time someone has lost weight or improved their performance in the gym, they beam with pride and joy.

The curious thing is all of these people were happy regardless of their current condition. They could still be very overweight, but dropping even a single inch off their waist made them feel fantastic. And who can blame someone for jumping for joy after they do their first pull up?

This was always in stark contrast to the individual who couldn't help but feel depressed over hitting a plateau even though they were already very lean, or the countless emails I receive from people frustrated by their performance, even though they are far stronger than most other people. All of these experiences have taught me that people are happiest when making progress towards their

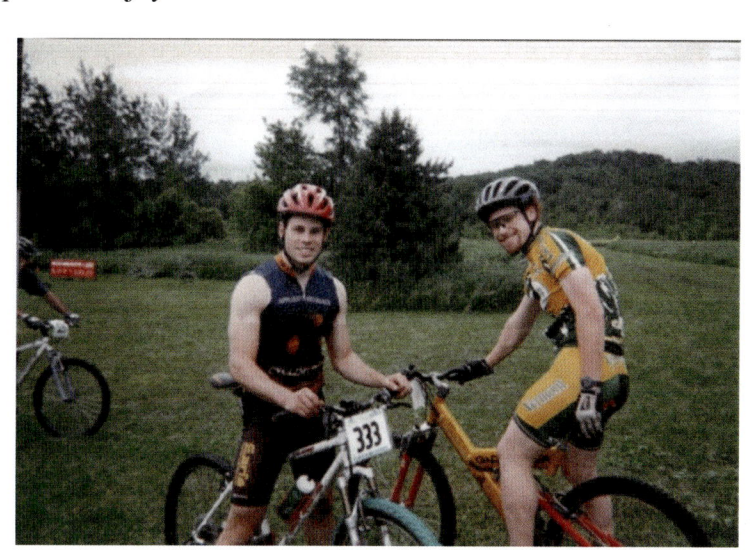

I was never the fastest bike racer, but beating my previous time always made me happy.

goals. It doesn't matter what their current condition is or how even how fast they are progressing. It seems all it takes to be happy is to be just a little bit better off from one day to the next.

Lastly, progression and consistency tend to build off of one another. It's much easier to progress when your habits are consistent. If your portion sizes are pretty consistent, it should be pretty easy to know if you're eating more or eating less. If your portions are all over the place, then it can be tricky to know if two slices of pizza are too much or not enough.

When you have progression, your motivation increases. As your results come streaming in it becomes much easier to maintain motivation and act with consistency. So consistency helps build progression and progression will help build consistency. Together, they create a whirlwind of momentum that can make getting in better shape seem almost automatic.

So now you have your first two action Delta Principles of progression and consistency. Next, you have what I call the personality Delta Principles; these are the ones that are more specific towards your personal beliefs and views of fitness.

Delta Principle #3 Logic and information

The next principle deals with the nuts and bolts of fitness. It's the actual science and facts of what makes the physical body change. The root causes are a good example of this as they deal with the basic science of what drives the changes in the body. Other examples include details about exercise programming, technique, and nutrition. I can't tell you exactly how to improve your golf swing while also telling you where you can get the best grass-fed beef in your state, but the root causes are a good foundation to start off from on your quest to fill in the details of how to fulfill those causes.

Don't stop learning

The biggest threat to the fulfillment of this principle is ignorance. You can only progress your habits to the degree you can execute them. If you never learn new information, you'll never progress very far regardless of how hard you work.
Consider running as an example. It's an exercise most anyone can do without any coaching or instruction. I know I sure didn't need any special instructions to run around on the playground when I was a kid. I even spent a short time on the track and field team in high school. Despite running for a couple of years before hand, but I was amazed how much I didn't know about running. I quickly learned that running around a track was just as technical as throwing a flying side kick through a stack of boards.

There is always more to learn, this is especially the case when it comes to basic exercises. No one knows everything when it comes to moves like push ups, squats and even walking. You could be the world push up champion, I promise you there is still a lot more to learn about how to push yourself up off the floor.

Delta Principle #4 Emotions and psychology

Simply put, your personal desires (wants, longings, and burning ambitions) are the driving force behind every choice you make in your healthy lifestyle. Whether or not you have that slice of cake or grind through another set boils down to the mental and physiological power you bring to the table.

Some claim your desires are an adversary that should be defeated or that desire guides you along the wrong path when it comes to getting in shape. While some emotions and desires can work against you, desire can also be one of the most essential, yet powerful aspects in helping you get what you want in life. If you decrease your desire, you'll cut off your motivational fuel line.

The idea of following your desire is a very misunderstood concept especially when it comes to fitness. One of the most common misunderstandings is that you either have the desire to do something, or you don't. This black and white thinking can lead you to believe you need to be highly motivated to take action. It can also lead some people to believe something is wrong with if they don't feel like doing something.

The truth is everyone has the motivation to both do and not to do something. No matter how fired up I am for a workout, or how much I want to order a salad when at a restaurant, there is always a part of me that would rather do the opposite. Just because part of you doesn't want to exercise or pass up desert doesn't mean something is wrong with you. It means you are human. It's natural to have even a little motivation against making healthy choices. This hesitation is mostly because healthy habits will always cost you resources. Your mind is always weighing the options between choosing to do or not to do something. It's part of having freedom of choice.

The key is to be aware of your motivation and the emotional foundation guiding your decision. There are always influences motivating you to hit the gym, just as there will always be reasons not to go. All of these influences are real, honest and legitimate. The question is, which influences are you going to focus on?

Acute vs. chronic desire

Acute desire is the type the experts warn you about. It's here one minute and gone the next. It's the quick and hot desire to eat too much pie or to skip out on the workout to hit the bar.

Chronic desire is much deeper, and while it doesn't always produce the white-hot flame that acute desire does, it's much longer lasting and more potent. It's the fuel that keeps your efforts going for years on end.

Here's a story to further illustrate the difference between the two:

Mountain biking is a sport often well suited for those with more courage than sense. During one particularly "fun" race, I was sitting at the finish with my friend and teammate, Chris. I was exhausted, hungry, and cold plus I needed to go to the hospital to stitch up my arm. "Chris," I said, "It's a good thing we love this bike racing stuff. Otherwise, you couldn't pay me enough to do this."

That race was a perfect example of the comparison between acute vs. chronic desire. I didn't like being out in the cold rain and crashing, but my deeper chronic desire to race my mountain bike won out. It pushed me through the momentary discomfort.

There most certainly will be times when you will have to fight your acute desires. It's the chronic desires you want to tune into that will give you the internal energy to keep moving forward. The key is being able to tell the difference between the two. In either case, the important point is that your internal desires are not hell bent on causing your diet or exercise habits to self-destruct.

It can be tricky to figure out what you want to do when it comes to diet and exercise. How can you tell the difference between your chronic desires and your acute desires?

One of the best ways to know what's best for you is to look into what activities you've enjoyed when you were younger. Did you like riding your bike or were you tumbling around in the backyard? Did you love steak and potatoes or were you more of a light eater during the day with a big heavy dinner? Our deepest chronic desires often create the long-term habits that originated in our youth and stick with us over the years. They are the hardest behaviors to change so why fight them when you can use them to your advantage?

If you liked being outside, then perhaps hiking or playground workouts are best for you. If you always felt best grazing all day, why try and force yourself to eat three big meals? Again, this is personal information that only you can know. You're the only person who knows, deep down, what you enjoy or dislike.

If you're unsure about what you like, don't worry. Your personal experience will teach you everything as long as you trust in yourself and keep your mind focused on what you want to accomplish. For now, it's probably best to avoid forcing yourself to do things you dislike. If you don't like yogurt, then don't force it into your diet. If you're not into yoga, then don't feel pressured to keep going to class.

The cost of fitness and how it relates to your motivation

Motivation is a term that's thrown around a lot, but few people study how to create it. Sometimes people believe you either have it, or you don't, and if you lack it then you need to get it as if it comes in a can from the store. You can't get motivation from a product or service any more than you can buy love or a strong work ethic. The key to motivation in fitness is in understanding the balance between the costs and benefits of your fitness habits.

Motivation isn't about a mantra you read on the Internet or receive in a speech during halftime from a coach. It's the result of a balancing act that's taking place on an emotional level. Imagine if you had a lousy job where you worked long hours for little pay in crummy conditions. Now imagine having your dream job where you only worked as much as you wanted and it paid over a million dollars a year. Which job would you be more motivated to continue?

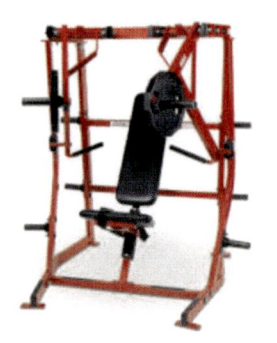

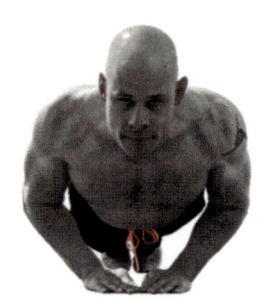

Compared to a bench press machine, the push up has a much higher cost to benefit ratio.

Motivation in fitness works the same way. It's all down to the ratio between lifestyle costs and the rewards you receive.

If your fitness methods bring you large benefits with low costs your motivation to practice those habits will be very high. If the lifestyle costs are high in comparison to the benefits, then your motivation will be low.

108

A lack of motivation is not a bad thing; It doesn't mean you're weak or lazy. When your motivation starts to dip that's the healthy reaction of your mind informing you the benefits you're experiencing are not worth the costs you are paying. Mother Nature knows you live in a world with finite resources. It's the universe's way of telling you you're better off spending your lifestyle resources towards something else.

How to increase motivation

Gaining motivation isn't rocket science. It's simply a matter of tipping the balance between your costs and benefits. The more benefit you receive from a habit and the lower the cost you pay to practice it the more motivation you'll have to continue using it. Here are a few examples on how to do just that.

Find your "whys"

Motivational coaches believe you should have a strong reason behind the work you do. Some people call this "finding your why." The idea is that someone with a bigger and stronger "why" will be much more likely to keep going when the going gets tough. Finding your why is simply another way to say, find your benefit. If you have a big enough benefit to chase after you'll discover more than enough motivation.

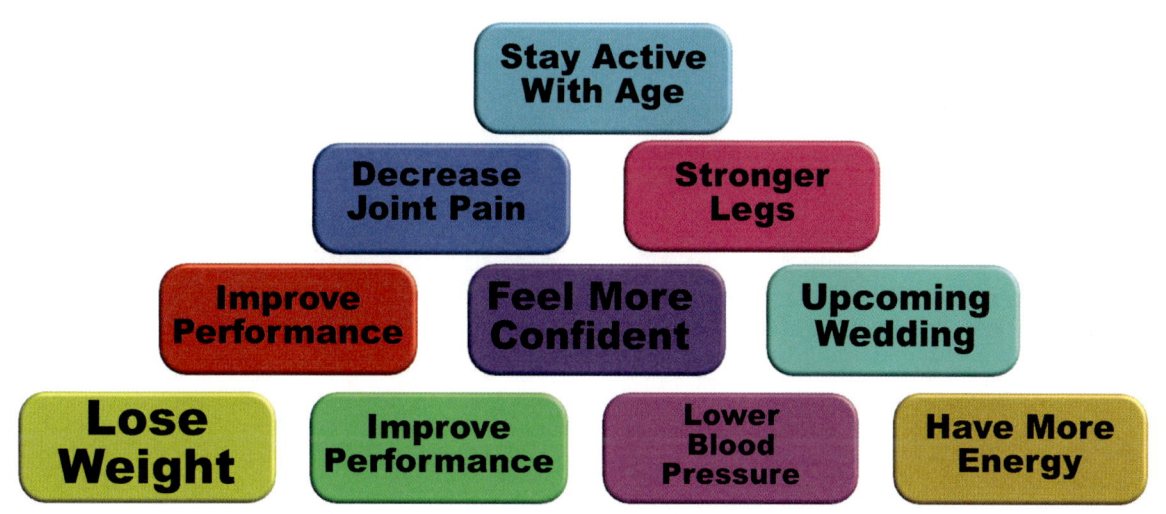

Motivation can come from a single big "why" or many smaller ones. Either way, it's important to focus on what matters most to you.

Personally, I've never had a big "why." What I have enjoyed are many smaller "whys." While none of them are big enough to motivate me on their own, all of them create a foundation of motivation. Having many sources of motivation works well because whys come and go. Even the biggest reason to do something might erode over time. Having many smaller whys will motivate you to keep going through the natural changes of life.

Cut costs

Another way to improve motivation is to decrease the costs you spend. I like making fitness habits very efficient. It's why I do bodyweight exercises at home rather than work out at a big gym. My entire home gym cost less than a pair of dumbbells, and I can do a complete workout within 10 minutes. Compare that to the costs of a monthly membership at a gym that's a 20-minute drive away.

Don't fall for the myth that spending more money or time will motivate you to "get your money's worth." Your mind doesn't care if you've invested a lot in the past, all it knows is what you're spending now and the benefits you're currently receiving.

Become better at what you do

Aside from cutting costs, the other way to increase motivation is to improve your proficiency in what you do. When you get better at doing an exercise or keeping a habit, you gain more benefits from doing it. This is what happened to a buddy of mine named Nick. One day he came to me complaining how much he disliked exercising his back. I gave him a simple mission, to focus on nothing but pull ups for two weeks. At first, he hated the idea. "You've got to be kidding me, pull ups are my least favorite back exercise of all!"

After two weeks he came to me all excited. "Dude, it's like I've thrown a switch! Now all I want to do is pull ups!"

Nick's story is not uncommon, and it perfectly mirrors my experience in almost every athletic activity I've done. From my Taekwondo-Do to push-ups I've always slugged through one workout to the next until I would cross some threshold. Suddenly my proficiency in that activity would skyrocket, and I would become obsessed with practicing it.

I'm not saying this is going to work for everything. Sometimes you'll try something for a while, and no matter how good you get at doing it you'll never grow much of a desire for it. That was always the case for me and running. However, if you're struggling to find motivation for a new activity you may just need to stick to it a little longer and get better at doing it. Once you do, you'll reap more benefits from the same amount of work and your motivation for it will grow.

Find your internal roadblocks

Nothing makes it easier to move forward than taking off the brakes, and almost everyone has some degree of psychological friction preventing them from moving forward. Most of the time, this is due to an emotional barrier that's preventing them from taking action. It doesn't matter what you know about proper nutrition or healthy eating. If you emotionally equate healthy eating to deprivation and stressful restriction, you will have a very hard time doing it on a consistent basis. You can have the perfect workout plan, but if you grew up making fun of gym rats, or even people who worked out, you probably won't make much use of your gym membership.

Sometimes a mental barrier can involve holding onto a habit as opposed to pushing one away. For example, you might find a lot of comfort in a nightly bowl of ice cream. Maybe you relish the Friday happy hour where you drink a lot with your friends. In either of these cases, it doesn't matter what I tell you from a logical perspective. I can tell you how fattening excessive alcohol consumption can be, or why exercise will improve your muscle tone, but It won't matter. The best physical science in the world doesn't stand a chance at motivating you to change if your mind remains stuck on old perspectives.

Delta Principle #5 A plan of action

All human accomplishments, from building the great pyramids, to baking cookies has only been made possible because someone created a plan of action. I used to rally against having a plan under the mistaken belief that a plan would force a structured use of resources. I thought "how can someone have freedom in a fitness lifestyle if they have a plan telling them when and how they should exercise?

My experience is very common, especially in fitness. Many people wobble between a strict routine and "winging it." Both approaches are extreme and lack one of the critical foundational delta principles. When you have a strict routine, you lack the flexibility to accommodate the natural flow of life. You also run the high risk of lacking progression. I often witness folks in the gym pick up a routine, and they stick with it, with little to no change for years on end. Sure they have consistency, but the lack of progressive change in the plan means lack of results.

On the other end, you have a total lack of a routine, and you make up your workout or diet as you go along. While this does give you a lot of flexibility and change, you'll lack any consistency to anchor your habits down.

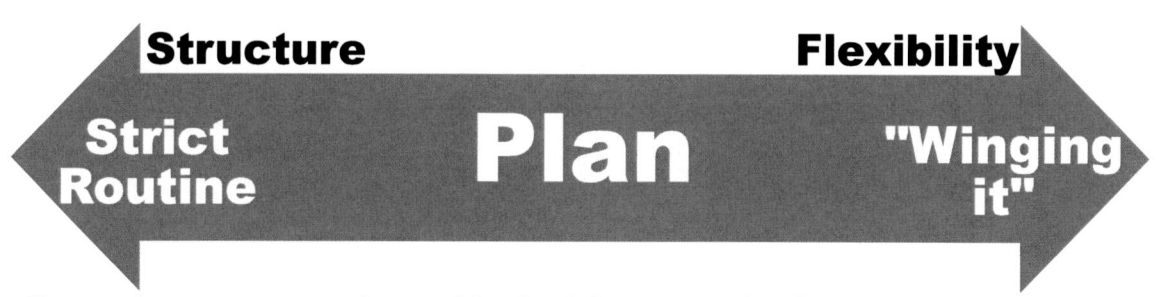

Too much structure can rob you of the flexibility you need to flow through life. Lacking in structure will make consistency and progression almost impossible. A plan is a mix of both.

The plan is the middle ground. It provides structure for consistency along with flexibility for progression. A plan is different from a routine because you're always free to change up the plan as needed. If your schedule changes or you go on vacation you still have your plan; you just adopt it to your new circumstances. If your current plan is to jog 3 miles twice a week, but you develop shin splints, then you switch to cycling for a similar amount of time.

While a plan offers the freedom to make changes, you only make a change if it's required. You don't make a change for any old reason. In the example above, you're switching out running for cycling due to injury. If that injury doesn't happen, you stick to running.

Getting started with a plan

I get into more detail on planning your fitness later on, but the best way to get started is to take a few minutes and draft up a simple weekly plan on paper. It's essential for you to write down your plan. Never trust your success to your memory. Write everything down because your memory will fail you at some point. Don't worry about figuring out the perfect diet or exercise plan. You don't need the best plan in the world. Heck, you don't even need a *good* plan. It just needs to be *a* plan, any plan at all you can execute on a consistent basis. Don't worry if it has a few flaws. Your success won't come from the plan you begin with, but rather the progression your plan develops over time. Your plan will go through many changes over time (as it should), and it's those changes that matter in the long run. Just keep in mind you'll never know what those changes should be until you take action.

So there you have it, the 5 Delta Principles that guarantee success. To help put it all together, I created this simple graph

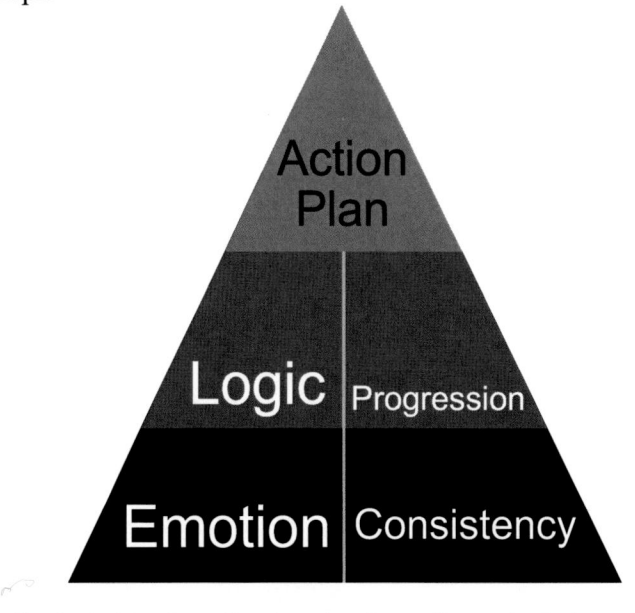

The 5 principles that will make or break your fitness. Apply them wisely.

This image graphically represents how all of the principles relate to each other. The foundation of the graphic consists of both consistency and emotion because these are the two foundational principles upon which everything else is built. Emotion and consistency also go together because your emotional drive is responsible for keeping your habits consistent for extended periods of time.

In the middle, you find the principles of progression and logic. Your progression builds upon consistent action, and logical learning is learned and utilized for emotional reasons. Progression goes with logic because learning more and working smarter is the primary source for most progression.

Finally, at the top, you have your plan of action which is built to use your personal emotion and logical knowledge to employ consistency and progression towards the cause of your goals.

I encourage you to print out this graphic and post it where you'll have easy access to it. You can find it on my website (www.reddeltaproject.com) it is a road map towards helping you get out of plateaus and challenging times on your fitness journey. Consult it on how well you satisfy each of the principles. It's a quick and easy way to troubleshoot any fitness program.

L and E dominance

Most people tend to possess either logic or emotion dominate personalities when it comes to their fitness. Since both of these principles are critically important, identifying if you're dominant in one or the other can help you target weakness that hold you back.

To put the emotion and logic principles into context, think back to the analogy at the beginning of the book where reaching a fitness goal is like traveling to a physical destination. Emotional drive represents the propulsion and fuel that moves you forward. Logical knowledge is the controls of your vehicle and the route you need to take to reach your destination as quickly and efficiently as possible.

While both emotion and logic are essential, neither one will get you very far without the other. If you have a lot of emotional drive, but little knowledge about what you are doing you just end up running around in circles. If you know the best route, but lack emotional drive you sit still and don't make any progress. Let's look into each of these in more detail.

Emotional dominance "I'll get results if I can just work hard enough"

People who are emotionally dominant have a lot of motivation and desire to take action. They typically don't wait until Monday to start the new diet, nor do they figure they will get to the workout when they have time. Instead, they make their habits a top priority and they get to work as soon as possible.

Since emotion is associated with consistency, they don't have a hard time to sticking to healthy habits. Lifestyle obstacles rarely slow down an emotionally dominant individual. It doesn't matter if they are on vacation, or if the boss asks them to work late. They will still find a way to get in their scheduled workout. It's for this reason that emotionally dominant people tend to stick to a plan or routine for a long time even long after they have hit a plateau. Their work ethic and persistence is unmatched.

The fault with the E dominant individual is they place too much faith in hard work. They take solace in the false belief they'll achieve success if they can just work hard enough. To them, the answer is simple, just work more, work harder and spend more resources.

The weakness of the E dominant individual is they sometimes don't know where they are going along their fitness journey. If you asked them what they need to learn or improve upon, they usually wouldn't have an answer for you because they lack the progressive knowledge from the logic principle. Part of this is because they don't know

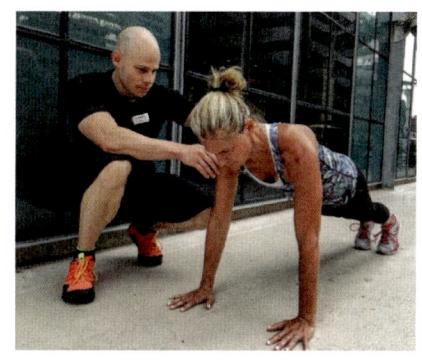

Hard work is important, but it won't get you very far without learning progressive information.

what they don't know. They are unaware there is more to learn beyond a few technical points in doing a push up. They don't know they can improve their diet beyond simply cutting out a few select foods. The other reason is they make assumptions about the potential to learn more. If they come across a book or lecture about fitness they assume they already know what the expert will tell them. For these reasons, the E dominant individual can work their tail off for months; even years and hardly make any progress beyond their "newbie gains."

Logic dominance "I'll get great results once I find the right program or diet for me"

The logic dominant individual possesses a lot of factual knowledge and technical know-how when it comes to the scientific facts behind fitness. They may own dozens of books on diet and exercise and subscribe to many blogs, magazines, and email newsletters. They are also perpetual students taking classes, asking questions and looking into the latest trends. Google is their best friend, and they can pick apart scientific studies with a fine tooth comb.

The fault of logic dominated individual is they place too much faith in learning the "right" way to eat or exercise. They are driven by the idea that there's always a better program or plan out there, so it doesn't make much sense to take action until they find it. They'll sometimes claim they can't get the results they want because they haven't found the program that works for them. Other times, they may claim they are waiting for a life event to finish a big project at work or when they can save enough money to afford to take action. They are constantly in a state of preparation, learning as much as possible to ensure everything is perfect before starting their plan. L dominant people are also more easily derailed and find it harder to stay consistent with a plan. If an obstacle falls across their path, they are likely to become discouraged and "take time off" rather than find a way to continue taking action.

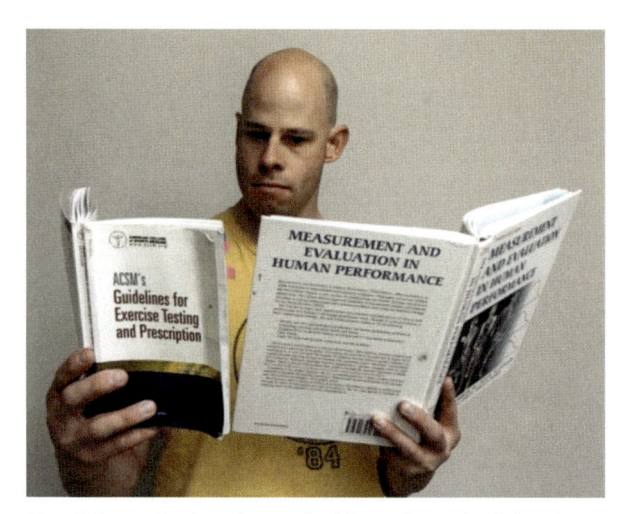

New information is only as valuable as the action it inspires.

The weakness of the logic dominant individual isn't a lack of know-how, but rather a lack of know-why. They may have a few psychological road blocks and have an emotional drive that's counterproductive to the habits they need to take to reach their goals. It may be something small, like feeling uncomfortable in a gym setting or something much deeper, like overeating to pacify the pain of an abusive childhood. In any case, the issue isn't a lack of scientific know how. It's from neglecting some internal friction that's making it difficult to apply that information.

Both logic and emotional dominance are weak, wasteful, and costly

Being emotionally or logically dominant can cause you to waste a lot of lifestyle resources while struggling to make much progress. Being emotionally dominant and motivated without a progressively improving game plan will cause you to roam around burning up resources. On the other hand, being logic dominant means you're spending a lot of resources learning and gathering information, but all of that information goes to waste without consistent application. The unfortunate thing is, both sides of the coin appear to offer the promise of great results if you can just spend more resources to either take more action or learn more information. This false promise only further motivates you to keep wasting your resources towards habits that no longer influence your cause.

The only solution is to bring balance back to the personal principles so you have both consistent emotional fuel and progressive information. Once you do this, the progressive information you learn will vastly improve the quality of your habits, so you don't need to spend nearly as much effort making up for lack of quality. At the same time, general fitness and fat loss aren't rocket science, and you'll be surprised just how far a little science can take you when you've applied it in a consistent plan of action.

Why people make fitness far too difficult and complicated

Balancing out your emotion and logic dominance not only saves you resources, but it also makes fitness a much simpler and easier endeavor. I know I sound like a late night infomercial when I write this, but I swear it's true. Fitness doesn't have to be nearly as difficult or complicated as most people make it out to be. It's easy to see why we believe fitness is so complex when you observe the false ideal between both logic and emotionally dominant personalities.
The emotionally dominant person over-relies on hard work so they feel like they have to push themselves to their absolute limits to achieve success. Since they lack the scientific information, they over rely on how hard they are pushing themselves and jump to the conclusion that reaching great results requires a super high level of work.

On the other hand, the logic dominant person relies on learning as much as they can. They look at all of the formulas and information involved in reaching a fitness goal and fall for the idea that getting in great shape must be akin rocket science.

It's these two personalities fueling the idea that fitness is a massively difficult and complicated thing to do. Sure it does take hard work, and yes you need to learn the science behind what you're doing, but both personalities tend to take it too far. The emotion personality believes you have to work yourself to death because they lack the information needed to make much progress with a faction of the effort. The logic personality believes you need a ton of technical know-how just to program a workout and cook dinner. Once the emotionally dominant person learns more, they can ease back on their workload and take it a bit easier. Once the logic dominant person applies some consistent action, they find just how far they can go with even the simplest of approaches. Combine the two together and you get a simpler, easier, fitness game plan that produces results.

Which personality are you?

Most everyone is either emotion or logic dominant, and your personality can even change from one to the other over time. The key is to recognize which personality you hold so you can begin balancing yourself out.

Maybe you've already recognized one or the other in yourself. If your plan is to work as hard as possible as long as possible, and you already know what you're doing, then you're probably emotionally dominant. Another sign is if you've ever told someone "I'm doing everything right, but I'm still not getting results."

If you've ever felt like you know what to do but you just have trouble doing it then you're probably more logic dominant.

Even your reaction to this book might be a good way to tell if you're emotion or logic dominant. Think back to when you were reading about the root causes. If you're logic dominant you may have thought to yourself "it's not that simple, there's a lot more to it than that." If you're emotion dominant, you may have felt like I was claiming getting in shape was much easier than you currently believe.

How to balance out emotion and Logic dominance

Once you've recognized whether you are logic or emotionally dominant, the next step is to break free of the false promise of just hard work or exhaustive research. If you're emotionally dominant, understand the key to your success isn't busting your tail until you drop. If you're logic dominant, recognize that you'll never find that program or information that will make everything work for you. Once you understand, deep down, that hard work or learning alone isn't the answer you can now begin to achieve balance by applying the habits on the other side of the equation.

If you're logic dominant, your next step is to start taking action on a consistent basis. Don't worry about figuring out the perfect plan or diet. Don't fret over the details just yet. All you need to know is enough information to begin putting your plan into action. Learning and acquiring information is no longer your top priority, taking consistent action is.

The funny thing is, once you start taking action you'll learn a lot more than if you kept your nose in a book. Nothing you ever read or watch in a video will replace the valuable information you'll gain from the experience of taking action.

If you're emotionally dominant, it's time to seek out how to work smarter rather than just harder. Look for some YouTube videos on what you're trying to accomplish or find a coach to look at your program. Even something as simple as asking yourself how you can better fulfill the cause of your goal by spending fewer resources can kick-start your mind to search for better information. You don't need to become a book worm and start attending night school to turn the tide. All you need is just one or two key take away tips from a book or blog to make a big difference.

The most valuable lesson about balancing out emotion and logic dominance is it doesn't take much to turn the tide. Just a little bit of consistent action will do wonders for even the most logic dominant individual. Reading just one book or even consulting a coach for 10 minutes can do wonders for the emotionally dominant athlete. This imbalance isn't something that takes a lot to turn around. A single breeze can turn even the harshest of storms around.

Part III: Taking Action

9: The Principle Governing Personal Change

Now that I've covered the most essential principles of Fitness Independence, it's time to start building up your action plan to apply them. After all, knowing the rules of a game isn't nearly enough to win; you must practice and master how you play the game itself. That's what this final section is all about. It's about putting the power in your hands and giving you the tools you need to be fit and live free for the rest of your life.

To start off, I wanted to explain the science behind how and why your body changes in the first place. After all, fitness is often about making changes you want or preventing changes you don't. It's funny; every expert has their theories on how to cause change, but very few people understand the natural principle that governs *why* your body either will or will not change. If more people knew the cause of physical change, most diet and exercise program would probably never see the light of day. Many programs ignore this principle and some even directly violate it all together!

The principle of personal change governs both your mental and physical state. It's not enough to change just change the mind or the body. Trying to change one without the other will only lead to frustration. If you want to change your body, you must change the way you think.

What is your attitude towards physical change?

What is your attitude towards your potential to make change happen? Some people try to fight the currents of change and exhaust themselves until they finally comply. Other's embrace change and want it to happen faster, or they try to steer it in ways that are not possible.

These various philosophies towards change in fitness can be liberating or enslaving. Some people perceive physical change as an inevitable thing, and there's nothing they can do to stop it. These are the folks who throw up their hands and claim circumstances like their age bring a host of ills from weight gain to muscle loss and take the position of a victim of nature. On the other hand, there are those who believe they're in control of their fate and can make anything happen. They seem determined to mold and manipulate their body as they see fit, and nothing is going to stand in their way.

As usual, the truth falls somewhere in between the two perspectives. For much of human history, people were ignorant of just how much they could train and condition their body. Outside of the athlete, most folks didn't know how to change or were uninterested in improving their body very much. With the explosion of our modern day fitness culture, people became aware of just how malleable the body is. If you wanted to look, feel and perform better, a few simple habits could make those things happen.

The thing is, once the train of thought towards physical change got rolling it took on a life of its own and expectations are now more based more on science fiction than reality. People started promising that it was possible to make outrageous levels of change happen within a short period and this over promising continues today as I've explored in the chapter on body building. It's time to set the record straight and get realistic about what is and is not possible with physical change.

Some solid facts about physical change

In my quest for reliable fitness answers, I've observed a few things about change that can be both liberating; yet help keep your feet on the ground.

1. **It's not so much about change but rather modification**

It's said that no matter what it eats or how it lives a bulldog can't change into a greyhound. The bulldog can become leaner, stronger or weaker but no matter what, it's still a bulldog. This idea hit home when I visited a car show showcasing some of the best modified cars in the world. Some of these cars looked almost nothing like what you would see on the street. The range of modification was staggering, but as I looked over all of those cars, a thought suddenly occurred to me. All of these cars were modified, but none of them became a different car. The Pontiac that was tuned for speed and handling was still a Pontiac. Sure it was faster and sportier, but it wasn't a Ferrari. Then there was the Camaro with the lift kit and big knobby tires. It would handle snow drifts better than a stock Camaro, but it would never be a Hummer or Snow Cat.

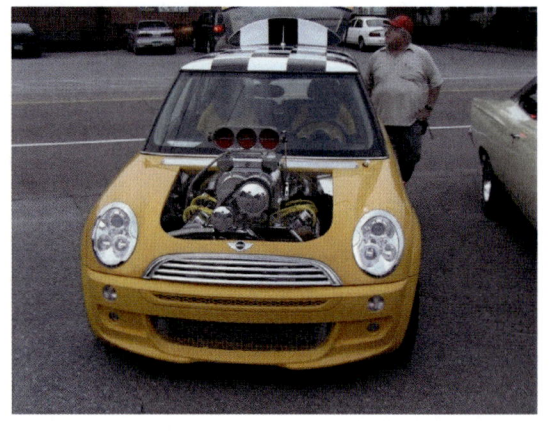

Even though this car is heavily modified, it's still a Mini Cooper.

The human body is very much the same. Throughout the years my body has made many modifications and alterations, but it has always remained the same general body. Sometimes I was faster and leaner and other times I was bigger and stronger. Throughout all of these phases, it never turned into a radically different physique.

2. **Bigger modifications require more resources**

There's yet another way in which the tuner-car analogy works. The cars that I was looking at in the show had massive modifications to them. Some of them had hundreds of thousands of dollars and countless man hours invested in those modifications. The bigger the modifications were the more resources were spent. There was never a quick and inexpensive way to massively modify a car.

The same can be said about your body. The bigger the change you're looking to make, the more time and energy it will require.

3. **You never lose the ability to modify your body**

No one has ever lost the physiological ability to adapt and change their body. It doesn't matter if you're 90 years old, you can still build muscle and strength. It doesn't matter if you're not a gifted athlete, you can always improve your performance. The ability to adapt is with you from your first breath to your last day on earth. What declines with age is the rate of change and how much total change can occur. So if you're a senior, I promise you still have the power to build muscle and strength just like any kid in high school. The same goes for fat levels. Age might slow you down, but it never grinds your fat burning furnace to a halt.

4. Change is somewhat unpredictable

Don't waste too much time trying to figure out how a new diet or workout will affect you. No one ever knows for sure what will happen once you change your habits. You can guess and come close, but there are just too many unknown influences at work to know for certain. The unpredictable nature of fitness is why it's so important to experiment as much as possible. You'll gain much more accurate information about the potential of a new habit through trying it out for a few weeks than you would if you sought to learn everything about it before taking action.

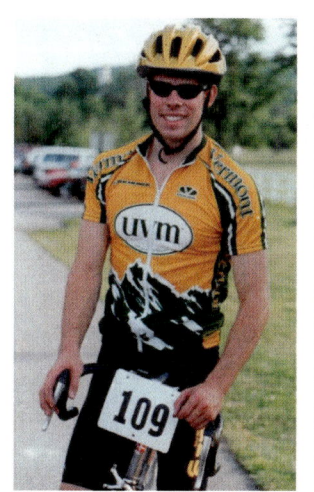

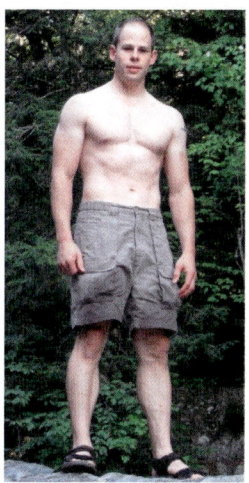

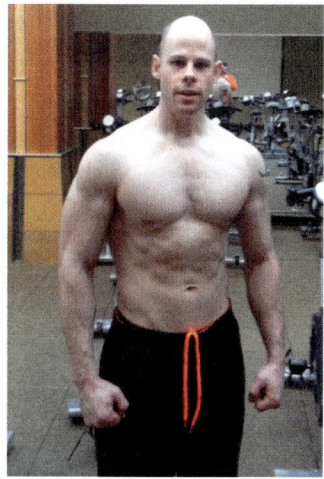

Some of the modifications my body has undergone over the past decade. Left, as a bike racer. Middle, a typical fitness enthusiast. Right, figuring out the Fitness Independence puzzle.

5. There are three aspects of change

There are three aspects to change when it concerns the human body:

- Change can happen quickly.

- Change can cost fewer resources and come fairly easily.

- Change can be big and very noticeable.

All three of these outcomes are possible for any goal you pursue. The only catch is that all three of them are not possible at the same time. At the most, you can choose two of those at the expense of the other. With that in mind, you have the following options.

Big & fast change that comes at a high cost

You can have change that's big and quick, but it's going to be very costly and difficult. A good example of this path is the popular fat loss reality TV shows. Contestants experience a level of change in a few months that would take most people years. This massive and rapid change comes at a high price. They often sacrifice all of their time and energy towards just getting in shape. They even give up contact with their friends and family. As far as lifestyle resources go, they are spending as much as they can which means little is left for anything else during the transformation.

This sort of change is ideal for those who are looking to make a large change happen as quickly as possible. Examples might include getting ready for an event like a competition or a social occasion like a wedding. It can mean a lot of change in a short period of time, but it's very difficult to sustain the change due to the high cost.

Easy & quick change that's not very drastic

The second option is you can have change that's relatively easy and quick. The cost is that it won't be very large or noticeable. This is the most common result a lot of people experience when they first get into fitness and that was certainly the case with me.

My first venture into fitness was a simple push up routine that I would do before bed each night. At first, I could hardly manage 8 pushups, but within 2 weeks I was doing 20 at a time. My routine involved little cost, just a single set of pushups each night that's all. The improvements were also fast as change was noticeable after a week or two, but no one was coming up to me and telling me how fit I looked. I was the only one who noticed anything happening because the change was slight.

Big & easy change that takes a while

You can cause change that's big and relatively easy, but it comes at the cost of time. This is the path I often advocate. It means making small, manageable changes that eventually add up to produce big results. The only thing is it takes time for those small changes to add up. Even though the fast and radical changes make for great TV, I believe most of the common fitness success stories follow along the slow-and-steady path. Whenever I run into someone who's come a long way their story is very predictable. They start off with small manageable steps like going for a walk during lunch or cutting back on desert. Often, these initial habits are not made in an attempt to make anything radical happen, but rather just to make some simple improvements.

Even though those improvements might be relatively small, they are enough to give a shot of momentum towards the next small step and then the next. In many cases, these small steps are made with a lot of time in between them. I started working out with just a push up routine. It was at least six months later until I stepped up and borrowed a set of dumbbells from a friend of mine. Taking small and manageable steps means the power of habit can firmly take root in your life. This makes it all the easier to take the next step.

Changing in small steps is in contrast to someone rushing into a fitness plan hoping to make change happen as quickly as possible. Much of the time, folks understand that the cost will be high, but they often underestimate how high the lifestyle cost will be, or they overestimate how much benefit will come about. Without the driving deadline of a specific event they look at the high cost they are paying and their motivation tips away from maintaining the habits. By contrast, the slow and steady method produces rewards that seem to come at a more manageable cost.

All three of these paths have their pros and cons and it's best to select the one that's best for your current needs. Also, bear in mind that you don't have to commit to one path of change forever. You can start off with a high-cost plan to jumpstart your progress and then shift gears to maintain your progress and keep moving forward at a more manageable pace after a few weeks.

Homeostasis; The cause of personal change (or the prevention of it)

Now that I've covered a few lessons about change in fitness it's time to get into the cause of *why* you may or may not change. That cause is a principle known as homeostasis.

The term homeostasis comes from the Greek *hómoios* meaning to be similar and *stásis* meaning to stand still. The dictionary defines it as the tendency towards a relatively stable equilibrium between interdependent elements. In the case of fitness, it represents the relationship between the environment you live in and the condition of your mind and body.

You might not run across the word homeostasis in the gym or while reading a fitness magazine, but you have probably run across a simpler term for it; *balance*.

Balance is a word that's often used with admiration within our fitness culture. Many fitness philosophies aspire towards a sense of balance between everything from the cells of the body to the balance between mind and body. Understanding balance is necessary, but it's not always a peaceful and harmonious situation. Balance can be one of the worst things for you, especially if you want to make progressive changes in your life. To understand why, it may help to start off exploring what balance means from a few different perspectives. The most obvious place to start is with Mother Nature.

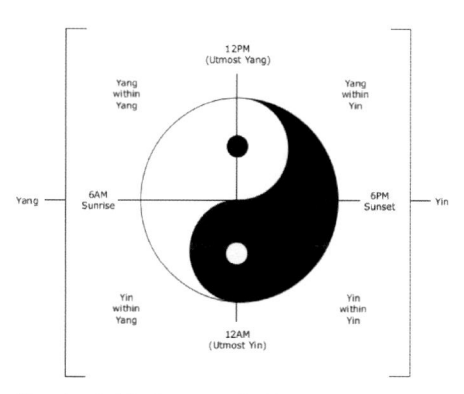

The classic Yin Yang symbol is a representation of balance and harmony.

Many ideologies, from ancient traditions to new age science, support the idea that everything in nature exists because of the ability to maintain balance. Day and night, high and low, hot and cold, everything exists because of a balance between dual forces. Even natural disasters like earthquakes and hurricanes can be explained by a pressure building up and then returning to a balanced state.

As far as the physical body is concerned, balance means survival. Animals that maintain homeostasis within their environment survive. Creatures that can't adapt to a change in an environment don't survive or procreate. The same is true on both a micro as well as a macro scale. Cells that are not able to maintain homeostasis die off in the body. If an entire species can't maintain homeostasis, it will go extinct. It wasn't an asteroid that killed off the dinosaurs; it was the environmental fallout from that asteroid that prevented the dinosaurs from reaching a state of homeostasis within their environment.

From a physical fitness perspective, balance means continuity. It means stability and the ability to stay the course. In other words, maintenance in whatever state you're currently in. If you're strong, you stay strong. If you're lean, you stay lean. It helps to keep you healthy, but the law of balance can work against you as well. If you're fat, you stay fat, and if you're weak, you stay weak.

Lastly, from a mental perspective, a state of balance means comfort and normalcy. A state of mental or emotional homeostasis what is often referred to as your comfort zone. When you feel like things are in balance, your mind is facing conditions that feel normal. It doesn't matter if those conditions are healthy or not. If you're used to smoking three packs a day trying to quit will throw your mind out of balance. If you're normal routine includes a hearty breakfast and a 2 mile run sleeping in and fasting until noon will feel off kilter.

So balance means survival, stability, continuity, and comfort. Its no wonder balance is painted with such a rosy picture. But that's only good if you want to *maintain* the condition you're in now. If you want to change something about yourself or your life, balance is the last thing you want to embrace.

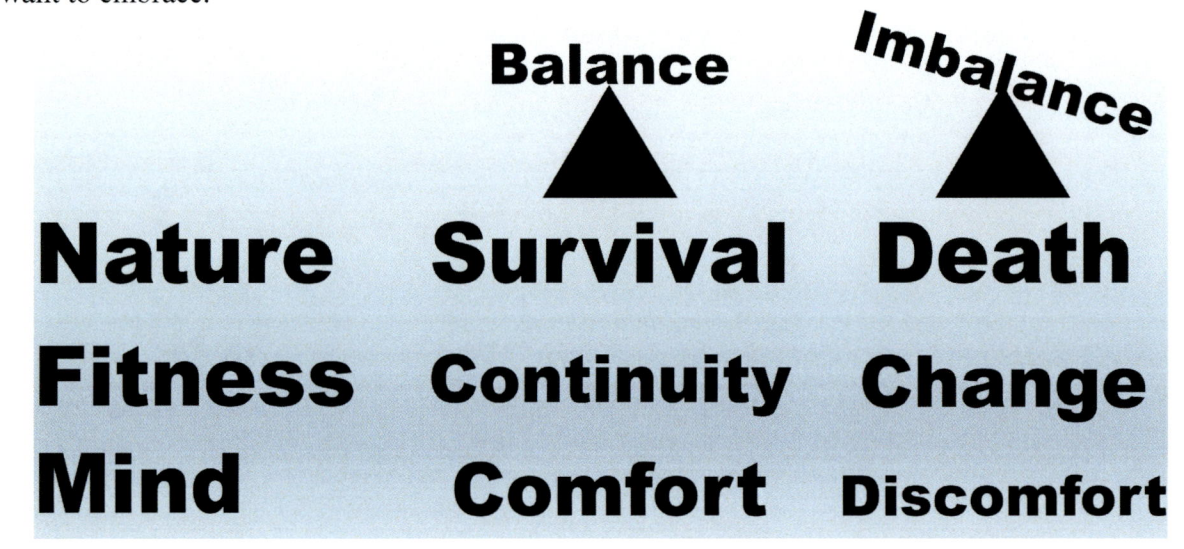

	Balance	Imbalance
Nature	**Survival**	**Death**
Fitness	**Continuity**	**Change**
Mind	**Comfort**	**Discomfort**

The natural laws of change can yield some pretty substantial rewards or penalties depending on how well you follow them.

Once you understand the principle of balance and homeostasis, you have the infinite power of Mother Nature at your disposal. If Mother Nature can use homeostasis to create or destroy entire galaxies, imagine what that power means in your quest to get in shape! But don't underestimate that power. It can both help you grow and progress or degrade and destroy you. Use it wisely through understanding the following:

1. **Homeostasis causes change**

Homeostasis is all about a relationship between you and your environment. Your environment could include fast food or farmer markets. It might involve pull ups or a night of drinking. If something changes in your environment, then your relationship also changes. When you and your environment don't quite match up, something becomes a little out of balance.

It's this sort of discomfort or stress that stimulates personal change. It's through these changes that you can regain homeostasis. Every change you desire, from fat loss to a faster sidekick is for the sake of returning yourself to a state of homeostasis.

2. **Homeostasis can prevent change**

Just as homeostasis can cause change, it can also prevent it from happening. Once again it's about a relationship between you and your environment. If you're in balance, there's no real reason for any change to take place. You won't lose weight, build muscle or grow calluses on your hands; there's simply no need to.

3. **Homeostasis isn't about good or bad, or healthy and unhealthy. It's about normal and abnormal**

Many theories believe the human body seems to know what is best for it and will gravitate towards healthy habits when given the chance. On the other hand, some folks talk about our caveman genetics as if we're hard-wired to lounge around and store as fatter as possible. Both of these perspectives completely ignore how the homeostatic relationship between you and your environment can be conditioned through repetition.

The body is capable of adapting to a wide range of conditions. Because of its highly adaptive nature, it's certainly possible to change to become comfortable with unhealthy habits. You can also become deconditioned towards healthy ones as well. Homeostasis doesn't cause or prevent adaptation for the sake of an ideal, but rather for survival within a given environment. You can set up your body and mind to be in homeostasis while eating lots of vegetables every day. You can also set yourself up to be in homeostasis with heavy drinking and smoking.

Knowing this gives you the power to understand that just because something is comfortable that doesn't mean it's healthy nor does discomfort mean something is unhealthy. It also protects you from misinterpreting a comfortable or uncomfortable scenario which happens all the time especially when it comes to diets.

It's very common for a fad diet to use the laws of homeostasis to convince you that certain foods are bad and other foods are good. This is done through asking you to refrain from eating certain foods for a period of time. After this "cleansing phase," you're invited to indulge in the "bad food." Predictably that food causes all sorts of issues like nausea, bloating, and it just might not taste very good. This discomfort is often mistaken as proof that the food is unhealthy for you and you always felt that way before but you just never noticed. It can sound convincing, especially when you don't feel very good, but it's a classic example of misinterpretation. The negatives effects aren't because of some dietary demon. It's because you're now deconditioned to handle that food.

I can make the same case for exercise. I challenge you to give up your favorite style of training for 6 weeks. At the end of 6 weeks, return to your preferred method of training for a hard workout. I'll bet anything you won't have the most positive experience. You'll be tired and achy and probably feel some mental discomfort as well. Both the physical and mental discomfort doesn't mean the workout is bad for you. It just means you're a bit out of shape for it.

4. Mental and physical homeostasis can get out of sync

Ideally, the conditioning of the body and the mind are in sync with one another, but sometimes things can become mismatched like in the case of addiction. The mind is craving something that the body can't handle very well.

A good example might be if you sustain an injury from working out. Before the injury your body felt invigorated and refreshed and the mind felt the pleasure and stress relief from the training. Then one day you feel a nagging pain in your right shin at the end of a run. The next day a dull ache radiates up and down your shin, but you pay little heed to it. The next day, you go for your usual run and the pain gets worse even though your body is telling you to take a break. You struggle through the pain because your mind craves the habitual run. You start masking the pain with painkillers and ice but eventually you concede and go to a doctor.

Your fears are confirmed as the doctor says you have a stress fracture that will take a several weeks to heal. It turns out the stress of your new warehouse job has been adding up over the past three months, and your new 10K training program was the straw that broke the camel's back. The law of homeostasis kicked in and was trying to pull you back to a manageable level by creating pain in your leg. It's Mother Nature's way of saying "you're taking on too much. Slow down." The only problem is your mind still wants to run even though your body doesn't. At this point you have a homeostatic conflict.

Do you stress the mind to comfort the body or stress the body to calm the mind? This mind and body conflict is possibly what originated ideas of "you vs. you" and "you are your worst enemy". Your mind wants one thing, but your body wants another. A homeostatic conflict is not something you can win. It's a losing situation, especially when your body is taking a beating. Every conflict is different but most of the time allowing your mind to make a change is the best course of action. In the case of the shin splint there's not a lot of wiggle room. The best thing to do is to find mental comfort through another outlet. It's often easier to change the body than it is to change the mind. The body is just a physical machine that is highly adaptive and receptive. Most of your systems run on complete autopilot. Things like that shin splint will heal just fine; you just have to stand aside and not interfere.

The mind is not so simple. It's the seat of your beliefs and emotions which are where your decisions are made. So even though your body may be trying to do one thing, your mind may override that signal. Maybe you insist on running for the relief of mental stress. Many people might keep going out of fear of gaining weight because they won't burn as many calories if they stop running.

Whatever the case, a homeostatic conflict is often the friction that makes fitness so darn difficult. The body wants one thing but the mind wants another and they are locked in a tug of war. When one wins the other loses. The best solution is to get both the mind and body on the same page.

Achieving mind-body balance may be one of the best things about Fitness Independence. Through focusing on the cause of your goal, you have many ways to accomplish your goals without feeling like you must stick to a specific plan. So if you're feeling the need to distress after work, you can take a long walk or try that Tai-chi class your friends have been raving about. If weight gain is your mental concern, then you can adjust your calorie intake or find another way to spend calories like swimming.

5. You can't win a homeostatic conflict, you'll either die or go crazy trying

One of the worst aspects of our fitness culture is the love of a homeostatic conflict. For some reason, having the body and mind in a tug of war is a sign of being tough and macho but a homeostatic conflict never produces long term progression. It does just the opposite as the tug of war weakens you in an attempt to get you back in balance.

If one side starts to gain the upper hand, then the other side will be driven into poor condition. In the case of the mind getting the upper hand severe physical damage may occur, and even death can result in extreme cases. This is why people die of eating disorders. The mind is so strong that it overpowers the physical signals the body is sending and eventually the lack of physical homeostasis results in the death of the individual. In less severe cases (like trying to exercise through pain) long term or permanent injury may result.

Mental breakdown can also happen as people put themselves under so much mental strain that their priorities become skewed and may resort to extreme behaviors like drugs or violence. When the mind is stressed, all bets are off and even the most insane or destructive behaviors can make perfect sense.

6. You must plateau at some point

It's a myth to expect your body to consistently make reliable change towards any goal. Our fitness culture loves to promote crazy expectations like you should lose 1-2 pounds a week for months on end, or you should always add weight to the bar every workout. Due to these expectations, when a plateau hits the person believes something has gone wrong. A plateau doesn't mean anything is wrong; it's just the opposite in fact. Hitting a plateau means homeostasis is doing its job, and you've adapted to the stress you've imposed upon yourself.

Change requires challenging your homeostatic condition and you have a finite capacity to do that at a given time. You must return to a balanced state to recover and refuel both your physical and mental energy. If you don't, the stress will continue to mount, and Mother Nature will force the plateau upon you. You'll burn out, become bored, frustrated or just mentally tired of pushing yourself. Physically, you may get tired, sick or injured.

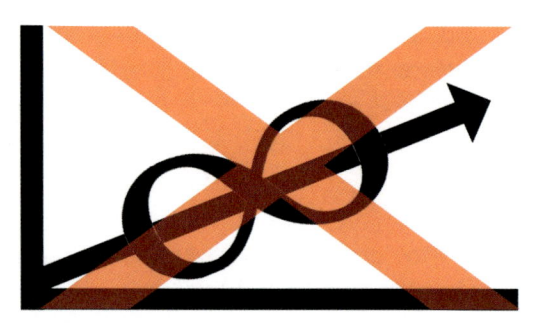

Your body wasn't designed to infinitely progress for long periods of time

There's a reason why all of these situations are making it harder for you to keep challenging your homeostasis. Mother Nature is trying to slow you down by force because you're not slowing down on your own.

7. Use homeostasis rather than fight it

The more you fight against homeostasis, the more you will lose. That's why I recommend working with homeostasis rather than fighting it. Instead of endlessly beating yourself up while expecting endless progression, you make a little progress and then purposely induce a plateau to hold your ground. When you do this, you avoid the pain and frustration that comes from being forced into a plateau plus you can maintain the progress you've made up until that point. Often, people will fight homeostasis until they "crack" and not only do they stop making progress, they fall backward and lose ground. This cycle is why a lot of people who lose weight on a diet, attempt to keep to the diet indefinitely. When they come off the diet, they regain all the weight they lost and even a few pounds more.

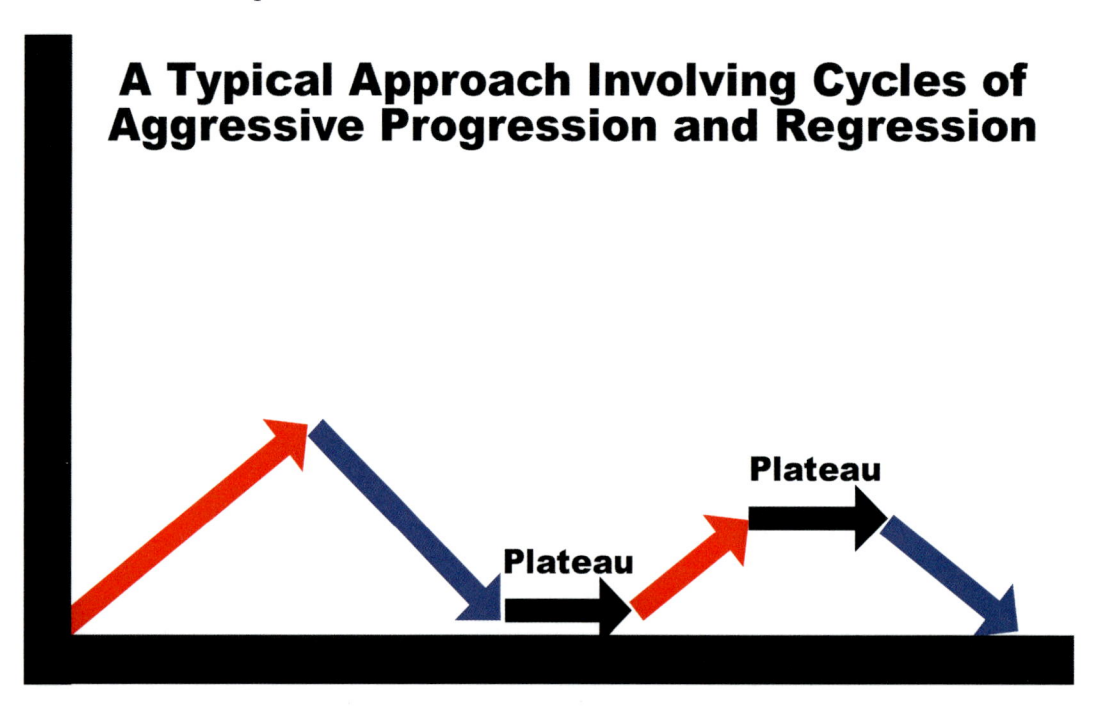

A Typical Approach Involving Cycles of Aggressive Progression and Regression

I like to think of change and homeostasis kind of like walking forward with a big rubber band around your waist. The overzealous folks will rush forwards as fast as they can and are pleased with the initial progress they make. Before long, the tension grows along the band and their progress slows to a crawl. They eventually stop and try to hang on for a few seconds, but they are exhausted and are flung backward to where they started. Once they recover from the setback, they build up the motivation to try and the whole cycle continues.

I propose a different approach. Instead of rushing forwards, make progress until you build up some tension. At that point, just hold where you are. You're not as far as your fast and furious friends, but you're playing it smart. You hold your ground and the band stretches a bit to let out some of the tension. When this happens, you move forwards a bit more, build up some more tension and once again hold and wait. After a few cycles of this, you notice your friends whipping back to the starting line, but you're still doing okay. You just stretch a bit, hold and move forwards once the tension loosens up. Sometimes that takes a little time, other times it might be a while longer. It doesn't matter though because you're not rushing forward. As your friends are in their latest attempt to rush forwards, you're already far ahead. To catch up they rush forwards, and they almost reach you until they are flung back again. Strange how they can hardly hold on to where you are because it's not that hard for you since you're getting used to the habits you've built up over time.

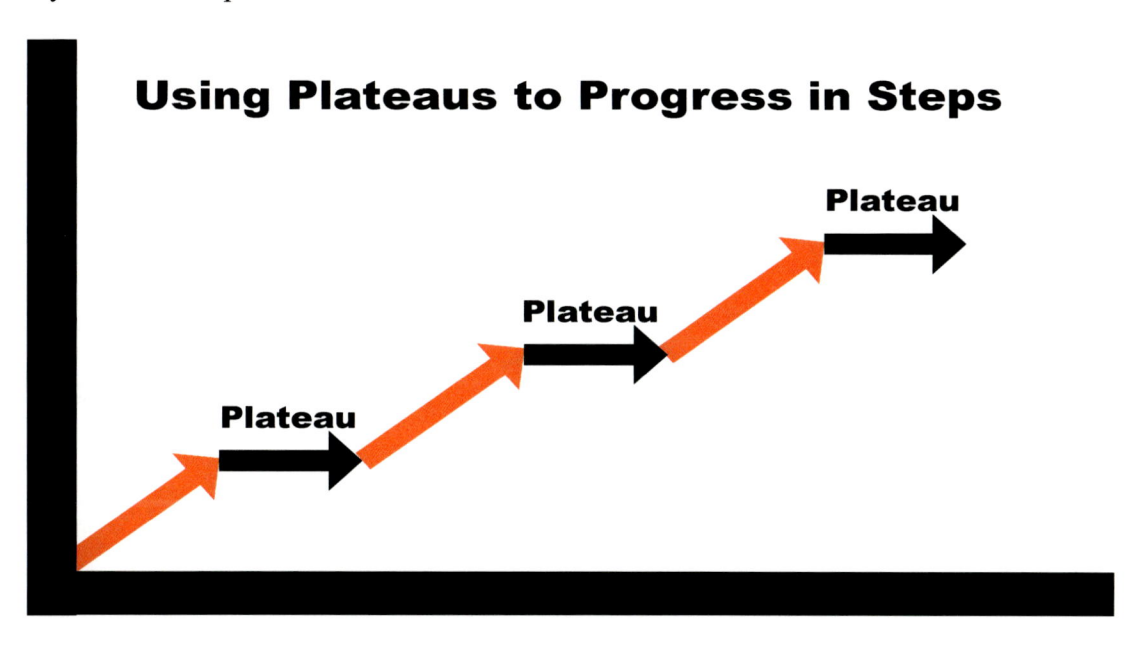

Using Plateaus to Progress in Steps

After a little while longer, you're much further than your friends have ever gone. They wonder how you did it. Maybe it's genetics or you're just somehow stronger. It's funny too because they can't recall you working all that hard for it. While they rushed ahead in a flurry of blood, sweat and tears you just plugged along at a modest pace. It's a mystery to them how someone could achieve the results you have, and maintain them, even though they are working so much harder.

This approach is the option of getting significant results relatively easily over an extended period that I mentioned earlier. The fast and aggressive approach is still great, just so long as you understand there will be a lot of tension generated very quickly. If you're working towards an event, this may be okay. Athletes do this all the time while understanding they can slingshot back a bit after the event. Keep in mind that this only works if there is a planned event and sometime afterward where you can regress back to recover. If your goal is to move forward and never come back, then it can be very frustrating to rush forward and fall back over and over again.

Here's a simple example; you're trying to lose body fat take a few days where you plan to purposely either increase your calorie expenditure or decrease your calorie intake. Let's say you plan on going on a 90-minute hike while having a light dinner each night. It's not easy, but that's okay you don't need to do it forever. It's just for a few days.

After the 3-4 days of your plan, you slightly increase the size of your dinner while no longer going on that long hike each day. You're now purposely holding your ground and trying not to eat too much, so you don't replace the calories you took out of your diet. You moved forward and then held your ground by proactively creating a plateau. Once you've held your ground for about a week, you can do it again and continue moving forward. With each round of cycling between a calorie deficient and a calorie balance both your body and mind become accustomed to the new level of body fat. It may not be a drastic change that happens quickly, but it is a gradual, more manageable, change that lasts.

The big lesson here is that progression isn't supposed to be linear. Expecting to endlessly lose 2 pounds a week, or do more reps each workout is nothing more than science fiction. Just as the seasons change in cycles, progress happens in cycles of change and plateaus.

8. Your environment is stronger than your willpower

The importance of taking care of your environment is highly underrated and underutilized when it comes to fitness. Many of the folks who struggle to control homeostasis are fighting against their surroundings. Your environment can include everything from the weather you regularly experience to the way your office is set up. If you have a bowl of your favorite candy on your desk, then you'll eat much more candy than if you had to make a trip to the vending machine. If you live right next to a 3-mile beach, then you're much more likely to go for a daily walk than if you lived in a congested, polluted city.

One of the biggest mistakes people make is trying to rely on their willpower to fight their environmental influences. They buy a big bag of candy promising themselves they won't eat too much. They purchase the membership to the gym far across town and vow to go there every morning before work. Like all forms of energy, willpower can be depleted and run low every day. It can be strengthened just like any other human capability, but it's never infallible. Sooner or later it always runs out.

Your environment is much longer lasting, and stronger than your willpower. That bowl of candy is on your desk all day every day. The temptation never lets up for even a second. So even though your willpower is strong in the morning, it wears down under the constant stress of denying yourself the candy.

Another example is to think of where your home exercise equipment is and where your TV and couch are. Most people keep their sofa and TV front and center in their living room. Meanwhile, they stash their hand weights in the corner of the dark, damp and musty basement. Under these conditions which do you think is going to be the most likely thing to happen after a hard day at work? Would you sit and watch TV all night or attack a workout in the basement?

I fully understand some changes in your environment may be tricky. It would be pretty hard to convince everyone in your family to build a gym in the living room and put the TV in the basement. Although, imagine what that would do for you! It can be hard, but every environment is subject to change. Last year I moved my TV into a secondary room. Without it always in the main living room, my couch and TV time plummeted without even trying. I also once had an apartment with a basement gym, but I stored a couple of kettle bells in the living room. Hardly a single day went by without picking up those weights and ripping through a few reps.

Homeostasis is immeasurably powerful. It can make incredible changes happen for you or it can keep you trapped in your current condition. It's 100% up to you to choose which will happen for you. In the next chapter, I'll lay out the steps you can use to gain more control over homeostasis and build a plan that will work best for you.

10: Building a Plan That Works for You

Things are wrapping up quickly here. You've got the basic principles of Fitness Independence, plus you even know about homeostasis the cause of applying those principles to control the changes you want or don't want.

Now it's time to start building your game plan. After all, you can't go into battle with the idea that hard work and persistence will win the day. You need to have a plan. It's the 5th Delta Principle that will lay down the foundation of your habits for your future success.

In all honesty, I've been a bit conflicted about writing this chapter. I've just given you the tools to understand fitness on a level few people ever reach. I've given you a ton of knowledge that makes you incredibly powerful, and yet, I would be taking much of that power away from you if I wrote out a plan telling you exactly how you should eat and exercise.

What sense does it make for me to write about the cause of fat loss and nutrition only to tell you how to eat right by following a strict meal plan? Why would I explain the cause of body sculpting only to give you a workout routine you have to follow to the letter? Doing these things would be like investing in 10 years of art school only to paint by numbers and connect the dots for the rest of your life.

If you would like a cookie cutter, run of the mill workout or diet, just do an Internet search, and you'll find hundreds of them in seconds. But I know you don't want cookie cutter and run of the mill. You don't want to risk your fitness results to some program created by a total stranger making random assumptions about what's best for you. What makes you think anything I write down here would be better than the guess-based programs you'll find online or in a magazine?

You're on your own

Fitness Independence means gaining the freedom and flexibility to achieve your goals as you wish. The only "downside" to allowing you this much freedom is it means you're on your own. Every choice you make is 100% on you. There's no sense in giving you the tools of Fitness Independence only to lock you into a program I make up based off of half-guess assumptions. If I did that, you would either go along with that plan, and it would be a poor fit for you, or you would recognize it as a poor fit, discard it, and be back to square one. You cannot be fit and live free while chained to a plan someone else made who has no idea who you are. Your best bet is to learn how to build your plan for yourself. You have to become your own best fitness expert.

Why you know best

When it comes to your personal fitness and healthy lifestyle you are the one who knows best. In fact, you understand a heck of a lot more than I do and every other fitness expert on the planet combined. I know that might sound kind of silly, especially in today's fitness culture. These days most diet and workout programs are built on the premise that you don't know what's best and that some doctor or personal trainer in Hollywood knows what's best.

Believe me, most experts, including myself; don't know what's best for you. Not by a long shot and here are six reasons why:

1. **No one else knows your lifestyle resources**

Your lifestyle resources are as unique to you as your fingerprints, and any diet or workout program must work within those resources. It's foolish to suggest you exercise for 2 hours every day when all you can afford is 30 minutes. It's idiotic to suggest climbing a mountain when you live in Kansas. You're the only person who knows what kind of time, money and energy you have to spend in the pursuit of your fitness goals. As such, you're the only one who can build a plan that won't strain your lifestyle resources and cause you a lot of stress.

2. **No one else knows your personal preferences**

Not only does your fitness plan have to fit within your lifestyle resources but it must also work within your personal preferences. I don't know if you love steak or detest the idea of red meat. Maybe you live for an easy jog, or maybe you prefer rock climbing. If you hate to run, jogging is going to be a poor match for you. However, if you get excited about the thought of riding a century or enjoy yoga, then those are methods you should pursue.

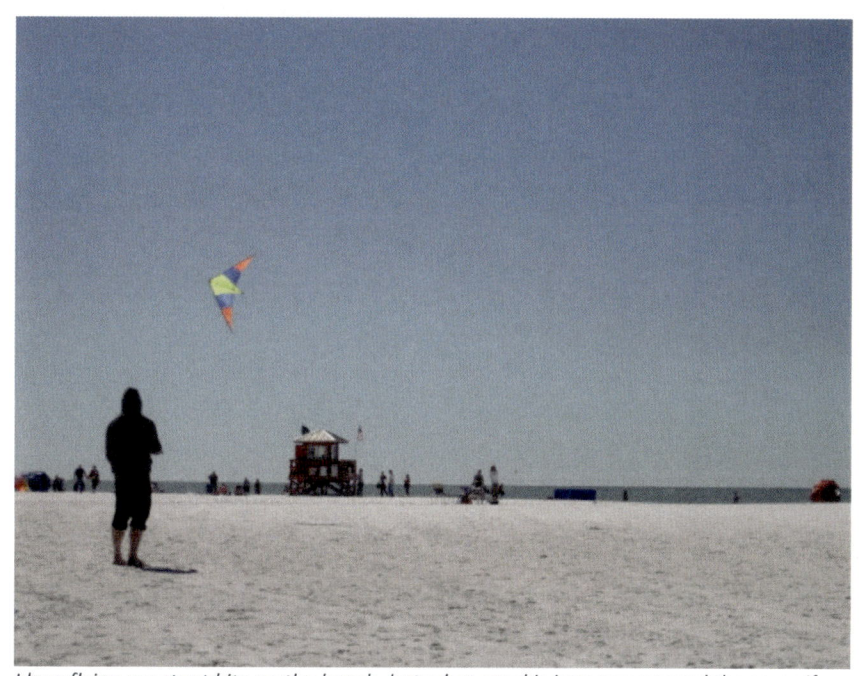

I love flying my stunt kite on the beach, but what good is it to recommend the same if you don't live near a beach or enjoy the sun?

3. **No one else knows about your surface influences**

Ultimately, your success boils down to how well you manage the surface influences in your life to fulfill the cause of your goals. No one else will ever understand your influences better than you. Unless I'm living with you 24/7, I cannot fully know how the influences in your life are altering your ability to fulfill the cause of your goal.

4. No one knows your vices, bad habits and hang-ups like you do

Being your own expert requires you to be open and honest with yourself. It means you can't keep telling yourself the same stories about why you can't reach your goals. You'll have to confront the habits that are holding you back. Once again, you're probably the only person in the world who will ever know your deepest secrets and shortfalls. Even if you depend on the advice of someone else, your bad habits will still sabotage your efforts if you try to keep them hidden. It's a lot easier to keep a bad habit hidden from a trainer you only meet twice a week, but it's a lot harder to hide it from yourself when you force yourself to confront them.

5. No one else cares about your results as much as you do

You're the one with the most skin the game. You have the most to lose and the most to win so only you will care the most about your success every single day.

I promise you your coworkers are not losing sleep over the 10 pounds you gained over the holidays nor is your workout buddy worried over why your knees hurt when doing squats. Sure, your trainer or coach will care enough to train you on the field or in the gym, but they probably won't call you on a Saturday night to make sure you are eating a healthy dinner.

6. No one knows what sort of changes you're going through

Your preferences, habits and surface influences change over time. You are the only one who knows how these things are changing and how they are influencing your fitness habits.

The only thing I, and anyone else, can know for sure is the cause of your goal. Other than that, all recommendations and programs are little more than an educated guess. The experts can give you a great start and a rough template to follow, but ultimately, you're the one who's in charge and has access to the vital inside information you need to build an effective game plan.

The death of self-sufficiency

As a kid, I was taught to do a lot of things for myself. If I wanted to get something done, I had to do it myself. If I wasn't motivated or disciplined enough to do something, it simply didn't get done. So when I started to get into fitness, I understood I was completely on my own. My success was mine alone to gain and lose.

I find this type of attitude sorely lacking these days. Now everyone needs someone to motivate them and hold them accountable. People hire trainers to build them programs and push them to do the work. They look up diet plans and workout plans telling them how to eat and exercise. Social media is filled with forums, clubs, and systems to support people. Not that social support is bad, but self-sufficiency is a skill set that's dwindling faster than the polar ice caps, and it's a damn shame. The more you come to depend on others for your success the less control and independence you have. Even though help from other people is great, the only way you can take control of your fitness is to be as self-sufficient as possible.

It's a shame such self-sufficiency isn't endorsed these days, but it's a downright tragedy that it's outright discouraged. Our fitness culture has positioned fitness as if it's rocket science that requires a Ph.D. and 25 years of elite level experience. Fitness is supposedly serious business, and it's not suitable for amateurs.

At the same time, there's this stupid notion that not only are you poorly equipped to make your own choices but you're probably doomed to fail if you do things on your own!

Many theories out there, especially concerning diet and fat loss, bring up this idea that people are programmed to be fat, weak and lazy. Through evolution, the human body was built to store loads of fat, move as little as possible, lose muscle and helplessly devour junk food while binge-watch Netflix.

If the eons of evolution have not screwed you over, the modern world surely will. Experts point fingers at everything from chemicals used during food production, to "addictive" processed foods, pollution in the air, and even your office chair is plotting to ensure you stay fat and weak. Only the experts have figured out the precise straight and narrow path you have to walk to save you from yourself and the modern world. Trust them, trust their programs and theories and above all, don't trust yourself. Just keep your mouth shut, your head down and stick to the plan.

Obedient ideas like these are not going to help you be fit and live free. Sure, you can force yourself to follow the leader, but why accept such limitations? Why not take back your personal control and rule your fitness lifestyle while significantly improving your chances of success?

Real self-control

The term self-control has been twisted and perverted to mean you need to conform to the demands made by others who supposedly know best. Forcing yourself not to eat what you want while choking down foods you don't like to eat is a good example. People love to boast how "good" they were because they ate right and didn't allow themselves to enjoy something. To them, they embody the essence of self-control, but to me, that's not self-control at all. That's obedience.

The way I see it, self-control isn't about being in control of you. True self-control is when your true self is in control. It about going after what you really want and doing things your way. You call your shots and learn what is best for you because who else can know you and your life any better than you?

Full control means full responsibility

Becoming your own expert can be both liberating and nerve-wracking. On one hand, you get to assume complete control over your destiny. You can do anything you like and call your shots.

On the other hand, taking full responsibility means looking at yourself in the mirror and knowing that everything is 100% on your shoulders. Every mistake and failure is on you. Then again, so is every success and victory.

When it comes to fulfilling the root causes of your goals, you have always been, and always will be, on your own. No one else can say "go ahead and relax, I've got this covered."

I understand there is a lot of security when someone else is making decisions for you. Allowing someone to make the decisions might seem easier, but in the long run it will limit both your potential and your lifestyle freedom. No one will quite know what's best for you due to their lack of knowledge about your way of life. Despite this, our fitness culture has long claimed that you don't know better so you should just learn the lessons from the experts and do as they command. If you do what they say, then you're "being good." If you don't, then you're "being bad." It's not about what's actually good or bad for you personally. Being good is more about obeying rules and programs rather than what's truly best for you. This is what I like to call the obedience mindset and overcoming it is the first step to reclaiming your personal power.

The obedience mindset

The obedience mindset is possibly the most prevalent form of discipline within our fitness culture. Every year diet experts tell people not to eat certain foods and folks shun those foods regardless if they need to or not. The same goes for exercise. Coaches and trainers endorse programs and training methods students adhere to even if those programs don't fulfill the cause of their goals or are poor influences towards those root causes.

While obedience might seem easier and safer in the short term, there are a few drawbacks to over-relying on it.

1. **Lack of true self-control**

As I mentioned earlier, true self-control isn't about blind obedience or obsessive adherence to a set of rules. It's about knowing what's best for you and having the skills to make the best choice in your present circumstance even if it goes against the rules.

2. **Not learning self-reliance and the confidence to make your choices**

True self-control isn't something you can learn from a book. You can only gain it through experience. When you base your decisions on obedience rather than self-control you are turning your back on the opportunity to gain that experience and thus learn what truly is best for you.

3. **Lack of flexibility and the ability to modify**

It's no secret that change is always around the corner, but diet and exercise habits based on obedience turn a blind eye to this inevitable change. Following the rules often creates a strict and rigid dogma that doesn't bend when the winds of change start blowing. This leads to habits that no longer work for you. Sort of like insisting on always sticking to the same diet that helped you lose 20 pounds but now it's no longer supporting your marathon preparation.

4. Not being able to listen to your self and understand what's going on

The idea of fighting yourself is very prevalent within the obedience mindset. The best teacher in the world is your own body. Every action you take creates both physical and mental feedback. This feedback is some of the most accurate data you'll ever receive regarding your fitness. Adhering to a rigid system often requires you to ignore, or even fight, that feedback.

To break free of the obedience mindset you'll need a whole new approach to your diet and exercise habits. An approach that doesn't hold the false promises that everything will be okay if you can just stick to the rules someone else created. You'll need to make your choices based on your skills rather than the ability to simply follow directions.

The skill based mindset

Sometimes when someone tells me that I'm "lucky" I say I'm not lucky.... I'm good. The ability to view diet and exercise as a game of skill, rather than a set of rules to obey, is the key towards achieving Fitness Independence. It opens large doors to both higher levels of fitness along with more freedom and flexibility.

Luck is a myth in the mind of those who possess skill. It doesn't matter if they are a master chef, a pro golfer or a top level salesperson. The capabilities of these individuals have little to do with luck and a whole lot to do with skills they have developed over time. Fitness is no different. Everything from building muscle to achieving 6-pack abs is about becoming proficient with a wide range of practical skills.

You can't get in great shape through luck any more than you can get lucky and paint a masterpiece. There are just too many choices you have to make over an extended period to achieve success. Sure, some people are fortunate enough to be born with great genetics or grow up in a healthy environment, but even the best genetics and environment can fall short when healthy skills are not developed. Here are just a few of the benefits of seeking the skills of fitness rather than just working hard to stick to strict rules or dogma.

1. Unlimited potential

Everyone has an unlimited potential to develop a skill. Just think of some of the greatest artists, and athletes who continually strive to refine their abilities. No matter how proficient they become, the potential to advance is always there. This is in stark contrast to how well you can obey a handful of rules. The best you can do is to stick to the rules, and then that's the end of the line. Once you've rid your diet of the "bad foods" or do the workout, your resources are then spent to merely maintain the progress you've achieved up to that point.

2. You may not always succeed, but you will never fail

Just think of when you were learning a skill like riding a bike or shooting a basketball. You understood you were going to miss some shots or take a fall from time to time. It wasn't what you were after, but at least you knew it was part of the process. You figured you would do better on your next attempt. In fact, you *expected* to do better.

This perspective is so important when it comes to getting in shape. The obedience mindset demands that you can't make mistakes or fall from time to time. When you do inevitably make a mistake, it's seen as a personal flaw and something must be wrong with you.

When you understand that fitness is a game of skill you expect bumps in the road. You know you're going to miss, and that's okay. You just pick yourself back up and try again knowing that you're getting better with each attempt.

3. Every day is an opportunity to practice

The more you practice a skill, the better you get at performing it. If you practice the piano every day you'll be playing show tunes much faster than if you practiced once a week.
Fitness doesn't just happen during meal times or in the gym. Every flight of stairs you climb and bite you take is an opportunity to practice the skills of moving your body and eating healthy.

4. More skill = easier success

Staying in shape should become easier with time. Not harder. Remember when you learned to ride a bike? At first, it was all you could do to stay upright and turn the pedals. As your skills improved, riding that bike became easier. Now you can just jump on that bike and ride with a fraction of the effort.

The same thing happens with the skill of fitness. As your skills advance, you'll find it easier to maintain the level of fitness you once struggled to obtain. This is why some people can make staying strong and lean appear effortless. It's not because of genetics or luck. It's because they have spent years developing their diet and exercise skills to the point where staying in shape is as easy as riding a bike.

5. Higher fitness skills mean lower lifestyle costs

When I first got into fitness I "needed" every gadget in an entire gym. My workouts were long and required a lot of energy. As my skills improved, I've refined my workouts considerably. These days my workouts cost a fraction of the time and energy. I also don't need a full gym of expensive equipment. All I need is a sturdy pull up bar and a solid wall.

6. Skills make fitness fun and enjoyable

Our minds, bodies and perhaps even our very souls have an affinity towards skill building. You can see this when people have an enjoyable hobby. The more they improve, the more fun they have. This is why something like riding that bike can be a lot of hard work one day and a fun past time the next.

Everyone has a mixture of the skill based and obedience mindset throughout the day. No one is going to fall entirely under one mentality or the other. Your long-term goal is to shift more towards building skills rather than trying to stay obedient to dogma. When you start learning something new, it makes sense to have more of an obedience mindset since you're just starting to learn the ropes. Over time, your mindset should shift more to a skill based mindset as your capabilities outgrow the rigid rules of the old program.

Building up your skills in fitness is empowering, rewarding and liberating. The trick is learning how to build up the skills necessary for your goals yet fit within the requirements of your lifestyle. To do that, you'll need to take personal stock of the most essential components of an effective personalized fitness plan.

There is no "fix"

Experts love to say there is no quick and easy fix when it comes to fitness. This claim is only half true. There is actually a lot of "quick and easy" in fitness. Going for a 15-minute walk is relatively quick and easy. Keeping red light foods out of the home is a much faster and easier way to improve your diet than trying to resist those foods. So it's not the "quick and easy" that's incorrect but rather the "fix" that needs to change.

Our fitness culture has a lot of goods and services promising to be the "fix" you need. The idea is that if you're trying to lose weight, build muscle or just stay healthy there must be something you can do or buy that can fix the problem. The idea of a fix sounds promising, but it's not true. When it comes to the big goals like fat loss and improved performance there is no single diet, program, product or service that can "fix" the problem for you.

Accomplishing life changing results depends on changing many habits and influences in your life. There is no one thing you can ever do or buy that can adequately take care of the fitness issue you're struggling with. Even the root causes discussed in this book are not a fix because once you understand them, your issues won't be fixed. You still need to figure out how to best fulfill them in a way that works for you.

I know a fix sounds tempting. Promising you can lose weight or get in shape through a single program or product seems ideal, but it's not what you want. You don't want a fix. What you want is a *process* through which you progressively fulfill the cause of your goal. You want a process over a fix for the following reasons:

1. **A fix will only solve your problem**

Think of fixing your fitness sort of like fixing your computer. You have some issue you want resolved and hope a fix lays within something you do or buy. The only problem is solving a single problem doesn't get you very far in both fitness and life. If you fix an issue with your computer, you don't make anything great happen. All you do is get back to your original level of performance. You're not accomplishing anything wonderful; you're just eliminating something bad.

The same thing is the case with fitness. Why settle for removing a problem when you can go so much further and accomplish much more? When you embrace a fat loss or muscle building process, you open an infinite world of potential. Since a process builds your skills you can go far beyond just solving the problem you're currently struggling with. You can make incredible things happen as you continue to develop and grow. A process has no finish line, and that's a good thing. It means you can continuously make progress and get more from your fitness than just solving a nagging problem.

2. Fixes delay gratification

The ironic thing is fixes are sold under the promise of instant gratification, but a process is much more efficient at satisfying this need. When you look for a fix, you perceive your situation in black and white where you want to have something, and right now you don't. Therefore, you can't be happy until you find the fix to your problem which is supposedly out there somewhere just waiting to be discovered. Unfortunately, fixes always remain just out of reach. Every new diet and workout program entices you claiming to be the fix you've been looking for. You may even believe you've found it as you try it and make some initial progress. This "honeymoon phase" never lasts long and before too long cracks and flaws appear in the perfect plan. After a while, the fix stops becoming a full solution and you continue your search for that one real fix that will work for you. It's like the carrot at the end of the stick, and you're the donkey forever chasing after it.

Embracing a process isn't like this at all. It holds the promise of instant gratification and reward, but most folks fail to recognize it. As I mentioned in the section about progression, people are happier and more satisfied when they are making progress. When you adhere to the process of your goal, you can make progress right here and now. You can put this book down and clean your kitchen from red light foods. You can pull those dumbbells out of storage and get them ready to use in the living room. You can even step right out your front door and go for a walk. These are just a few examples of quick and easy ways to start on the process of satisfying the cause of your goal.

When you look for a fix, things, like going for a walk or excavating your home gym in the basement, might not seem like a big deal. They are not enticing because they are not a fix. Going for a single walk won't fix your weight problem. Setting up your dumbbells or even doing a workout won't fix your weaknesses. If you're looking for a fix, you probably won't look for little steps like these. You might brush them off if someone suggested them to you because they are not that fix you're looking for. The result is you never start the process of fulfilling the cause of your goal and remain stuck as you continue to search for that one elusive fix. In other words, the more you keep looking for a fix to your problem the longer you stay broken.

Once you recognize fulfilling the cause of your goals is a never ending process you can free yourself from looking for a fix. While there isn't a quick and easy fix, you can quickly and easily get started on the process of fulfilling the cause of your goal with these simple steps:

Step #1 Figure out what you want

Nothing significant ever happens until you know exactly what you want. The goal you set is your destination; it's the reason behind every choice you make. The better you know exactly what you want, the better you will know how to achieve it.

Choosing a goal just might be one of the hardest things you'll ever do on your fitness journey, but it's not something you should avoid. Everything you do from this point onward is about fulfilling the cause of your goal, and you won't know what that cause is until you know what you want. Always remember, your body adapts to the specific practical instructions you feed it. Your body doesn't understand what "being fit" or "being strong" is. It's like going to a restaurant and saying you'll have "whatever with a side of something else." Your body will adapt to the specific instructions you feed it, whether you know what those instructions are or not.

Some people find it difficult to define what they want. It may be because they aren't sure what they want, or they don't know how to put it into words. Others worry they might seem selfish to stand up and proclaim they want something for themselves. They might also be afraid of looking too shallow through asking for a goal centered on appearance. There's also the fear that once they set their goal, they are potentially turning their back on all of the other possible things they could go after. If they want to improve their bench press they might be missing out on "functional strength." If they put more emphasis on cardio, then their strength might suffer.

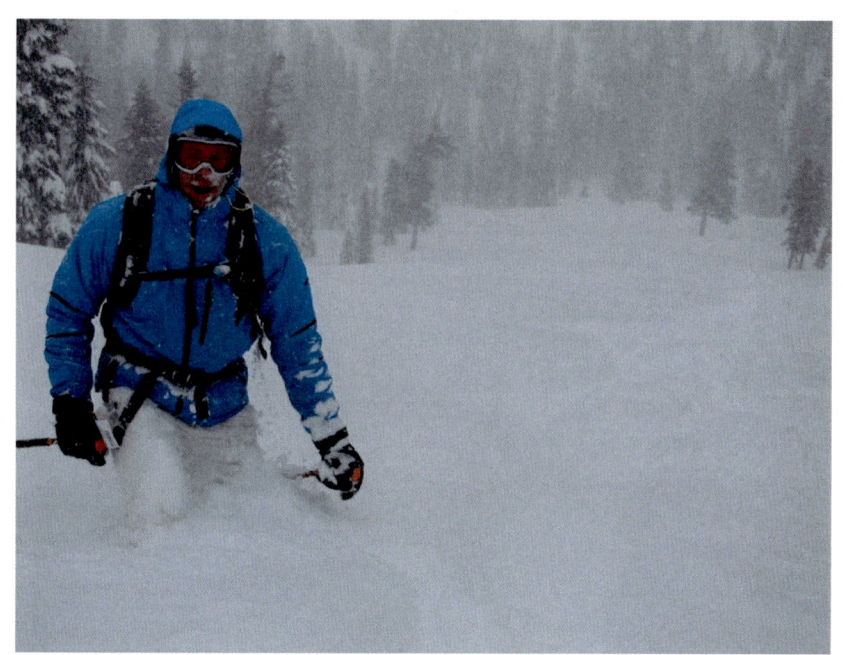

While cold and snow might not be everyone's idea of a good time, Its always been a goal of mine.

The second hardest thing about choosing a goal can be sticking to it. Our fitness culture loves to embrace a sort of fitness ADHD where people are constantly changing from one goal to another. All of this change results in switching various programs and their accompanying habits. While I don't want to discourage anyone from making changes once in a while, it's essential to pursue a single goal for a long time to achieve anything. As the saying goes, the man who tries to chase many rabbits often catches none.

Step #2 Become aware of your surface influences

Once you have your goals nailed down it's time to start observing the various influences that can both help or hinder your ability to fulfill the cause of that goal. If you're looking to lose weight, what influences do you have that impact both your calorie intake and calorie expenditure? If you want to build muscle, what can you do to increase time under tension? If you want to eat better, look at the food influences you come across throughout the day.
Once again, only you can do this. No one else can be sure about what your influences are and how they influence your goals.
This step can be a real eye-opener for some people. Once you have your sights set on your calorie balance or muscle activation you'll be amazed at how many influences are in your everyday life that you never actually paid attention to. Your daily habits will become a bit clearer to you, and every bite you eat or step will seem more important.

Step #3 Take stock of your lifestyle resources

While you're looking at your surface influences, you'll also need to take stock of your lifestyle resources. Just like shopping for a car, it pays to know how much you're willing to spend. If you can't devote 2 hours a day to working out, then take that into account.

I highly recommend staying well within budget when it comes to your spending. If you have an hour lunch break, plan a workout that takes 45 minutes. If you can spend $500 on a home gym, try to get everything you need with $50 to spare. Remember, the origin of most stress in life is when you're running against the limits of your resources. If you plan to spend a little less than you can afford you'll stand an excellent chance of having a plan that won't stress you out.
I know it can be tempting to spend as much as possible, to squeeze every minute you can during your lunch break or max out your credit card setting up your home gym. It's that whole idea that if you spend more, you'll get more in return. Don't fall for it! It might work a little bit in the short term, but always spending to the limit of your resources increases the chance that your short term habits will fail to produce long-term results.

Step #4 Start fitting resources and influences around your preferences

As I mentioned in the chapter on Delta Principles, we humans tend to do things because we *want* to do them rather than because we need to do them. We are emotional creatures and will use logic to justify our emotional choices.

Your emotions can either work for you or against you. Much of our fitness culture teaches people to fight their emotional tendencies, but I say why not use the power of your emotions to your benefit rather than a detriment? Maybe you don't like running, and maybe hiking is more your speed. You can burn loads of calories doing either activity. Maybe Yoga isn't your cup of tea, but you love kickboxing. Both can teach you balance and flexibility just fine. Unless your goal depends on doing a particular form of exercise, you're free to use whatever methods you wish.

It's also crucial to pick your battles. You don't have to make everything perfect to succeed. It's not uncommon for people to hit a stumbling block where they struggle to change one or two simple habits. They spend a lot of effort trying to get one little thing taken care of while neglecting the other habits that's a lot easier to change.

It's kind of like taking those multiple choice tests in school. The teachers always say if you get stuck on a problem then skip it and come back to it later. Otherwise, you might spend most of your time trying to figure out that single problem which is keeping you from the ones you can easily answer. The same is the case with fitness. It's just not worth the effort and resources to change one stubborn habit especially if it's a relatively minor influence. You may be better off leaving a couple of stubborn habits in place and focus your energy in other areas that can make a bigger impact with less cost and effort.

Step #5 Test

I get a lot of email from people asking me if a particular diet or exercise method will work for them. To be honest, I usually don't know any more than they do. No one ever knows for sure how something is going to work for them until they roll up their sleeves and get busy trying it out.

Some folks turn to endlessly researching a method they are considering before they invest their lifestyle resources into it. This can cause the person to spend far more lifestyle resources than if they simply tried the program.

Your experience is by far the most valuable fitness information you'll ever gain. You will learn more in 3 days of testing out a workout than in 3 years of reading about it and asking experts what they think. Once you know enough to try something, it's time to stop researching and start doing! It's the doing that will teach you what you need to know, not the latest magazines, blogs or bestselling books. All that stuff just gives you a starting line. Beyond that, you have to take your first step.

Step #6 Record and Track

The experience and knowledge you gain from trying something is invaluable, but many people fail to capture it. It's kind of like a fisherman on the side of a river just watching the fish swim past him. Your experiences are just like those fish. You need to have some way to capture them. This is why it's so important to keep a log or journal.

A log forces you to stop and think about your experience. Is eating a high protein breakfast making you feel good or sluggish? Are you getting stronger in your Yoga class? What are some of the frustrations you're experiencing from that new push up program? A log will remove a lot of the mystery in your plan, and you get to cut right to the chase of what's working and what isn't.

You can track anything in your log from your performance to how something tastes to you. Whatever you feel is important should be recorded. That said, it's vital you record data that's directly related to your goal. If your goal is to change your physical shape, then keep pictures of how you look and body size measurements. If you are trying to run faster, track how fast you cover a set distance. Don't focus too much on variables that are only roughly related to your goals. A typical example is when people track their weight, but they want to lose body fat. Sure, the fat on your body is an influence to how much you weigh, but both water and muscle are also an influence to how much you weigh. If you want to lose weight, track your weight. If you want to lose fat, track your fat.

Keeping a log might seem like a time consuming and tedious chore, but I promise you it will save you loads of lifestyle resources. Some people have spent thousands of dollars and years of time on habits that are not working for them, but they turn a blind eye because they are not tracking their progress.

Step #7 Modify

A lot of people skip from one program to the next in the hopes of finding that fix that will solve all of their problems. They try the latest trend with hope and excitement, make a little progress, but ultimately run into some challenges. These issues mount and the individual quickly hits a plateau. They are then trapped and feel like they are spending lots of resources just to maintain their meager progress. Usually, they throw the whole plan in the trash and end up back at square one where they started. After a while they find a new method to try and the whole cycle starts all over again. I like to call this the cycle of frustration.

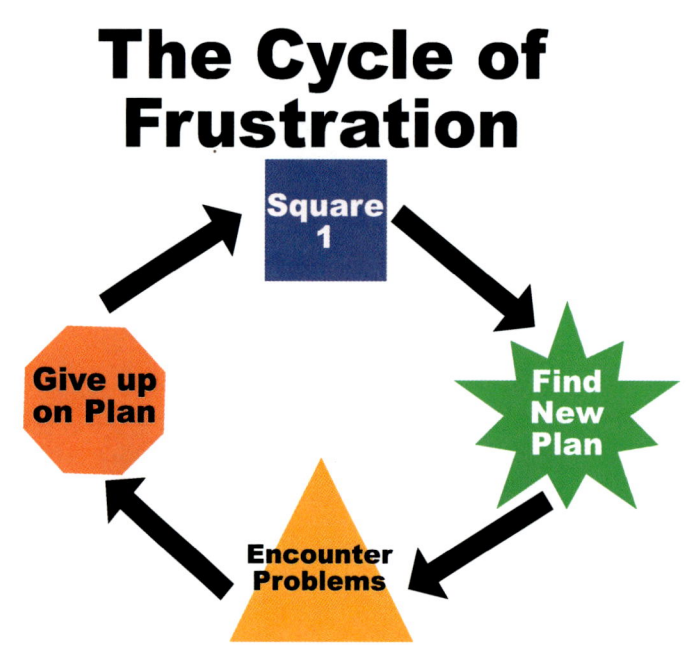

Don't throw out your plan, even if it's not working for you. Modify your program as you like, just don't give up!

The cycle of frustration is incredibly taxing both physically and emotionally. Each repetition is a roller coaster ride of ups and downs, but ultimately you just run around in a circle without going anywhere. It's also very expensive since each repetition requires starting your fitness program all over again with new startup costs. There are books to buy, courses to attend, experts to consult and a whole host of new challenges to overcome. This is why it's much smarter to avoid tossing out the whole program and making modifications to it instead.

No program is going to be a perfect fit right out of the box. There are always components that simply won't be a good fit for you. The good news is you don't have to keep all of those parts as a whole. Every diet and workout program is like a high-end suit you can endlessly tailor for a perfect fit. If you don't like a particular exercise in a program, you can swap it out for something else. If you find you can't go without a special food, modify your diet to include it. If you don't have time for a long workout, then make it shorter. You don't have to keep your plan perfectly intact at all times.

This act of modification is the ultimate solution on how to build a custom program that works best for you. It will fulfill the cause of your goals, so you make progress in the right direction. You'll mold the methods around your lifestyle resources so you can continue to afford to keep pursuing your goals. Most importantly, you'll adapt the program to your preferences so your motivation will continue to flourish. It's the ultimate win-win, and you never have to go back to square one.

Where should you start?

If you've been in the fitness game for a while you probably already have, or at least have used a plan before. If that's the case, then all you need to do is to continue with your current plan and make modifications to further fulfill the cause of your goals within your preferences and resources. This is especially the case if your current plan is working for you. One of the biggest mistakes I see is when someone is making progress, and they trash their entire plan for something else. When they do this, they are going from something that's working and taking a complete gamble on something entirely new. Every time you completely change your plan you're rolling the dice on your results. When you modify your program you're making a much more calculated decision so your chances of progress are much greater.

But what if you're just starting out from scratch? What's your first step? Simple, your first step is to find and try out a plan, any plan at all, that appeals to you and stands a good chance at fulfilling your root causes. Diet and exercise plans are all over the place. Most of them are free and easy to find on line. You can find them in magazines or on the Internet. Maybe someone you know has been following a plan for a while and would be happy to share with you what they've been doing. You can even make up your plan based on the experience you've gained from using various plans in the past.

I know it can be intimidating to look for and commit to a plan, especially when you're starting out. No one wants to pick an inferior plan. The good news is you almost can't fail when you're starting out. It's a myth that the beginner has the most to lose, but it's the opposite. As someone who's starting out, almost anything will be useful to some degree.

How to Build a Plan That Works for You

1- Establish What You Really Want

2- Seek Out Surface Influences

3- Take Stock of Lifestyle Resources

4- Fit Influences and Resources Around Preferences

5- Apply and Test

6- Record and Track

7- Modify Based on Experience

Lastly, keep in mind that your ultimate success won't come from the plan you start with. Remember, the Delta Principle that brings you results is progression. All you need from your initial plan is a place to start. Beyond that, the details don't matter. The plan you start off with isn't going to get you to your goal no matter how perfect it is. It's the plan your first program *progresses into* that will bring you what you seek. You don't need to understand every step of the journey. The first few steps as all you need to know. Once you take them, the next few steps will become apparent as long as you keep looking for them.

Why people never find what works for them

Like the Delta Principles, the previous steps are all required to find what works best for you. If you don't have a clear and defined goal, all of your choices from the start will be more a blind guess than a carefully aimed decision.

If you're not taking surface influences into account, you can go through your day oblivious to how your environment is controlling your homeostasis. This will make it much easier or harder for you to fulfill the cause of your goal.

Not taking stock of your lifestyle resources is a sure-fire way to run yourself ragged as you attempt to achieve too much, and you exhaust yourself. If you don't know how much you can afford, chances are you will go after something that's well outside of your lifestyle price range.

Fighting or ignoring your personal preferences creates an uphill battle you simply cannot win. The only way you'll ever stick to any change in behavior is if the new habits bring you more pleasure or satisfaction than the previous ones.

If you keep your nose in a book or on the web forum, and never take action, you'll never know how things are going to work out for you. No matter how much you learn, nothing beats the genuine and honest information you'll gain from experience.

If you don't track your progress, you'll never know for sure if something is working for you or not.

And lastly, being open to modification will allow you the freedom to build your methods, so they become a perfect fit for you in time. It will also ensure your program will adapt to the natural changes of your lifestyle.

Building your own program will give you power, flexibility and freedom over your health and fitness. It will allow you to control homeostasis to move in and out of your plateaus as you wish to create changes at will.

Don't sweat the details unless…….

A lot of folks get stuck considering every little detail of a workout routine or diet. They are unsure of what to do so they waste time "researching" even the smallest detail. Should they take a protein shake after their workout? What kind of protein is best? When is the best time to take it? Should they use milk or water? If they use milk is almond milk better than dairy? What about whole milk or skim? Some people get lost in the rabbit hole, never to see the light of day as they consider every possibility. It can create paralysis by analysis and prevent you from taking action.

Over the years I've learned that most of these details not that important. Most of them are too small to hold much influence over the cause of a goal. This is in contrast to a lot of the fitness information out there. Open up a magazine or watch the news and the hype is everywhere inflating the gravity of a single influence or some minor detail. Small influences are portrayed as being far more important than they are.

With that said, some details can make all the difference in the world. A slight shift in bodyweight can make knee pain disappear during lunges. Adding a few shakes of hot sauce can make a dish delicious. So it's not so much about ignoring the small details, but instead knowing which ones matter the most.

The best way to know if something is important is to experiment and find out for yourself. Stop looking for the answers on the Internet or in a book. If you're wondering if skipping breakfast twice a week will speed up fat loss, just make a plan and give it a try. This whole fitness thing is pretty hard to mess up. Chances are, you probably won't do anything wrong by trying out a different push up or adding a lemon to your water during your workout.

Here's how I look at it; "Don't sweat the small stuff unless the small stuff makes you sweat." Most of the time you'll give a tweak to your routine or diet and find nothing notable will come from it. In these cases, you're free to discard the influence or keep it depending on your personal preference. Maybe you keep the lemon in your water just because you like the taste a bit more, or maybe you ditch the protein shake because it's not worth the cost.

When you do stumble upon a significant detail, you should receive some pretty clear feedback from it. Maybe that small technical shift in your push up makes your muscles work much harder. Perhaps you feel nauseous with milk in your protein shake, but water is fine. These are the times when you certainly do want to make a note of the difference and act accordingly. You'll only know for sure what details are important through your personal experience. I can give you my ideas about adding milk vs. water to a protein shake, or how to breathe while doing pull ups, but I'm only basing those answers off of my own experience which isn't nearly as accurate as your own. Even the scientific research sighted in journals is just the experience of a group of individuals in a study. That doesn't make it invaluable, but it is still removed from your life enough to have limited application. So don't sweat the small stuff unless the small stuff makes you sweat and the best way to know if it does is to roll up your sleeves and get to work.

Doomsday and utopian thinking

Anyone can quickly become engrossed in the smallest details due to what I call utopian and doomsday thinking. This thinking is when various experts or media inflate small influences to appear much more significant than they really are. Open a diet book and the author pulls no punches when they write about how certain foods are evil poisons that will lead your health to ruin. At the same time, other foods or exercises are portrayed as a minor miracle in how beneficial they can be. The term "super food" is a good example of how something as simple as a blueberry is nothing short of a savior to the modern diet according to some experts.

Everyone has their bias and prejudices. When people talk about things they don't believe in their views can be colored with extreme negative perception. The same works with things they believe in and want to support. Their diet or exercise method is the best thing in the world, and you would be a fool not to follow it. Hence what they believe is unhealthy is a terrible thing that you should always avoid.

The doomsday and utopian portrayal of fitness methods are often supported by larger than life results. Supposedly whatever is bad can create untold pain and suffering while the proper methods offer an endless stream of rewards. For example, some claim eating a cheeseburger will make you fat, clog your arteries, impair your performance, stunt your growth, muddy your concentration, contribute to global warming, decimate the rain forest, enslave the poor, poison the water table, and make you a social outcast who's destined to be sad and alone for the rest of your life.

On the flip side, that new workout program will heal your wounds, improve your performance, make you hot and sexy, balance your hormones, improve mental focus, help you get into med school, kill cancer, cure aids, save the whales, and bring peace and love to the world. Imagine, the balance of hell on earth or a utopian society all depending on what you eat and training with the right equipment!

Of course, I'm exaggerating, but not by much. I've known people who blame their relationship problems off of what they eat and claim that their workout changed their life. I won't argue that diet and exercise can be powerful agents for the quality of your life, but I'm not about to start preaching that all of your problems will be solved with the right diet or workout plan.

The doomsday and utopian thinking is very dangerous. It throws the realistic expectations of fitness out of balance. That cheeseburger may be a significant influence towards many objectives, but it's only an influence. There's no guarantee that eating a single cheeseburger will cast you into a hell of fat gain and poor performance on the field of competition. At the same time, it's unreasonable to expect to be the star of the basketball team or to build the perfect abs just because you work out a certain way.

Many influences are important, but most of them are not *that* important. Knowing just how much influence a single habit holds is key in assessing the true potential it has towards fulfilling the cause of your goal. Doomsday and utopian thinking prevents this from happening. It makes assessing and choosing your habits sort of like being in a fun house where the mirrors distort the real image into funny shapes. What's big becomes huge and what's small becomes tiny. In some cases, it's reversed.

Honestly understanding the cause of your goal is like stepping in front of an actual mirror where you see everything as it truly is. Nothing is hyped up nor is it glazed over. Ultimately, the worst part of doomsday and utopian thinking is it doesn't give you control over your choices. You remain in a constant state of reactive action where you're trying to adhere to the best possible outcome or avoid a worst case scenario based off of what someone else believes. Your motivation is artificially created from a potential punishment or a promised reward both of which may be grossly over exaggerated claims for the sake of selling you a product or dogma.

What's even more confusing, is the science and understanding of fitness is always changing the doomsday and utopian landscape. One day food like, coffee is a terrible thing, and you need to avoid it at all costs and the next day it's a super food. Your favorite weight machine at the gym could be the best thing for your abs today, but a year from now it may be in a magazine article titled *The ten worst core exercises ever.* It's difficult to get an accurate bead on what's good for you and what isn't.

The new role for expert advice

As you continue your fitness journey, many experts will play various roles in your success. It might be tempting just to shut down and never listen to what any expert has to say, but that wouldn't be a good idea either. While a lot of expert advice is biased and prejudiced, it can also be very helpful in your fitness journey. The key is to look at it with a neutral point of view.

This requires reframing your orientation to the fitness experts. In many cases, the expert is seen as the one in charge, and you're standing before them asking them what you should do. I advise a role reversal. *You're* the one in charge. You're the one sitting on the throne as the king or queen of your fitness domain. When you need help, you call in the expert who can then offer ideas and suggestions.

You don't need marching orders to get in shape. All you need are a few ideas and suggestions. You then take those ideas and give them a test drive. Contemplate how that idea might influence your cause. If it doesn't seem to be much of an influence, then it might not be worth pursuing. If it sounds like something you might enjoy or benefit from give it a shot. Try it out, see what happens and note your reactions. From there, change and modify it as you wish to best fit your personal needs. Don't let the doomsday and utopian spin they put on their ideas cloud your thinking. Do what you feel is best, not what they claim is best. If the expert claims fruit is bad for you, but you gain benefits from eating it then listen to your results, not the expert's opinions. If they claim an exercise is pointless, but you love how it makes you feel, then keep doing it. You're the one in charge. You're the one who knows better. Not them. They are your advisors and nothing more. They can't tell you what to do; they can only offer you their ideas which can be very helpful. Just never forget that it's your actions, experience and reactions to those ideas that matter most.

11: Delta Fitness Methods

There are countless ways you can fulfill the cause of any fitness goal. One of the benefits of Fitness Independence is you get to get in shape on your own terms. You can eat, train and live how you want. If you want to work out on a $12,000 weight machine with a celebrity personal trainer, you can do just that. If you want to grow your own food and chop wood for your workout, you can do that too. You're free to do whatever you like.

While costly fitness strategies are perfectly fine to use, I'm a big fan of super-efficient methods that cost less and deliver big results. In this chapter, I want to introduce you to some of my favorite tools and methods that embody productive efficiency. I call these, the Delta Fitness Methods. (DFMs)

The Delta Fitness Methods all share a few unique characteristics:

1. **DFMs are inexpensive**

These methods are all incredibly inexpensive regarding time, money, discipline and effort. While no method is free of any cost, these methods often use a fraction of the resources used by other methods.

2. **DFMs are very effective**

While a lot of methods are cheap, very few can produce great results. Most of the cheap exercise gadgets you often see on late night infomercials are examples of this. While some of these methods hold some value, many of them are cheap products that produce inferior results. I've selected these methods because not only are they effective, but you'll probably find them to be more efficient than their costlier counterparts.

3. **DFMs must have low entry requirements**

All of these methods are as simple as plug-n-play. You hardly need to buy or learn anything to get started using them. They don't require a degree in nutrition or exercise science for you to start using and benefiting from them. Even if you're a complete newbie to the fitness game, you can jump right in and get to work. If you are unsure of what to do, you can quickly find answers through a quick Internet search.

4. **DFMs help you infinitely grow and progress your skills**

Even though these methods are easy to start with they also hold an infinite capacity for growth. This means that no matter how proficient you become with using them you'll always be able to improve how you use them and further fulfill the cause of your goal.

5. **DFMs fit your lifestyle and preferences**

Diet and exercise habits are supposed to fit within your lifestyle; not the other way around. These methods are all chosen because they are some of the most fun and enjoyable methods available. While you may not enjoy using all of them, I believe you'll find some enjoyment in at least a few of them. At the very least, they should improve your enjoyment of your habits making them easier to stick to and more rewarding.

Okay, let's jump to it!

First up we have the Delta Fitness Methods for exercise.

1. Progressive body weight training

No form of exercise embodies freedom, versatility, and skill-based results like bodyweight training. You don't need a gym membership and a body weight home gym only requires some open floor space and a place to hang from. It's also a great method for customizing things around your individual preferences since your own body is your equipment. There's no such thing as an exercise that won't be a good fit for you and your current level of fitness.

At the heart of bodyweight training is the essence of activity which is learning how to use your body better. It's a system for understanding yourself on a deeper level and that understanding can branch out towards any other aspect of your life.

As far as results go, it's a myth that bodyweight training will only take you so far. I used to believe that as well until I seriously started to study it and was surprised that I could gain better results through bodyweight training then with more equipment-based methods. Part of the reason is that bodyweight training has significant advantages towards fulfilling all of the Delta Principles. Its efficiency and flexibility make it easier to stay consistent with a workout plan as life becomes turbulent.

Single leg squats are a low-cost high-reward exercise.

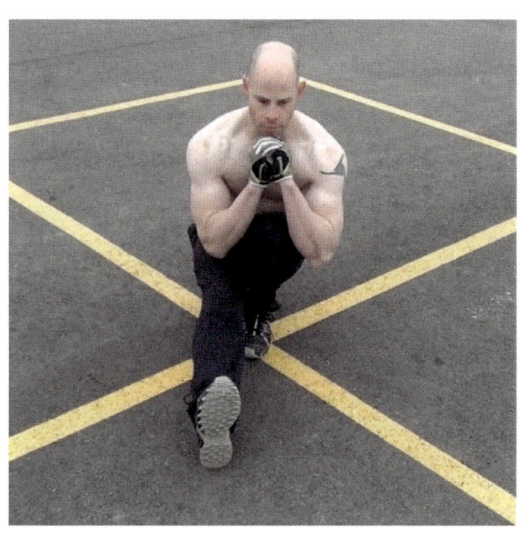

As far as progression goes, many bodyweight disciplines have an infinite degree of progression to fulfill any cause you desire. Also, bodyweight training uses what I call technical convergence which means it holistically requires numerous characteristics of fitness at the same time. As you seek to grow stronger with advanced exercises, you also improve your balance, flexibility, muscle control, and a host of other fitness characteristics. In this way, you progress in many aspects at the same time with a few select exercises. Lastly, engaging in activities that move you through space can be fun and enjoyable compared to just sitting on a machine and moving levers.

2. Walking, hiking, and running

Have you ever noticed how the cardio floor of your local gym involves doing exercises you can do outside for free? Almost all of the machines are designed to help people walk, run, jog, and hike which are activities humans have been doing long before the invention of the health club. Those high tech cardio machines don't give you the ability to exercise. They provide you with the capacity to exercise without going anywhere. It's perfectly okay to do stationary cardio, but it's important to understand that this type of exercise requires a lot more cost to you while also potentially decreasing your benefit.

Going for a walk is a prime example. To walk on a treadmill, you need to use a machine which costs a lot of money so you need to either buy the machine for yourself or you have to pay a monthly membership fee to visit a gym that will supply one for you. If you belong to the gym not only do you need to pay the dues but you also have to spend the time and energy to get to and from the gym and potentially have to wait for the equipment to become available during busy times.

It's also worth mentioning the mental discipline required to use the machine. Many treadmills come equipped with TVs in order to keep the user's mind occupied and prevent boredom. I've heard many people claim that they can run or hike outside for hours, yet it takes a lot more effort to do machine based cardio for even 15 minutes.

3. Riding a bike

One of the best fat and calorie burning machines ever invented is collecting dust in millions of garages right now. The humble bicycle is a wonder machine which gives you the power to enjoy the world around you while helping you get in fantastic shape. If you're trying to lose weight the bicycle is a great machine in helping you burn calories because it helps to support your weight. This provides you with a low impact exercise as you enjoy the sun on your face and the wind in your hair.

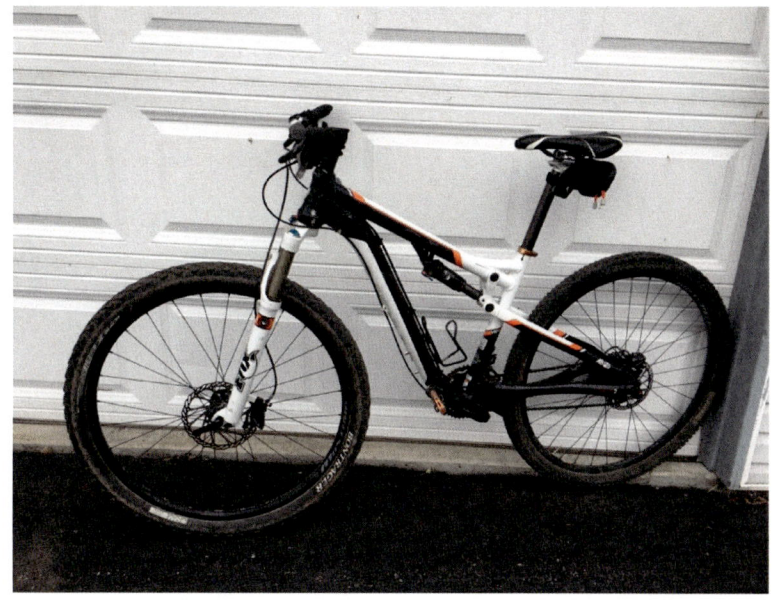

My faithful steed. Your bike doesn't need disk brakes or full suspension. It just needs someone to ride it.

Cycling can become a very complicated and expensive hobby with some bikes costing as much as a small car however it doesn't have to be so. From a perspective of health and fitness, there is no difference between the most expensive racing machine and a bike available through a local garage sale. As long as the bike is reliable and comfortable it serves as much promise as it can in fulfilling your fitness needs.

If you haven't used your bike in a while any bike shop can provide a full tune up for about the cost of a typical oil change for your car. It's worth it to ensure your comfort and safety.

4. Free Weights

Next to body weight training, a simple set of free weights can be a very inexpensive and versatile weapon in your training. All you need are a few simple hand weights and maybe a flat bench and you can duplicate almost any strength exercise in a fully equipped gym. Free weights are also low maintenance and can last a lifetime with proper use. Like bodyweight training, free weights are also a skill-based tool with a very low entry point. You can get started with using basic dumbbells today and spend a lifetime mastering the basics.

A word of caution though, as building a free weight home gym can quickly take on a life of its own. I've seen more than a few home gyms start off with some basic dumbbells only to grow into a room filled with clutter that cost thousands of dollars. When I built my own home gym, I quickly collected a wide variety of plates, bars, handles and accessories that filled every inch of my apartment. In time, I learned that while lots of toys and options can be fun, most of them are not necessary.

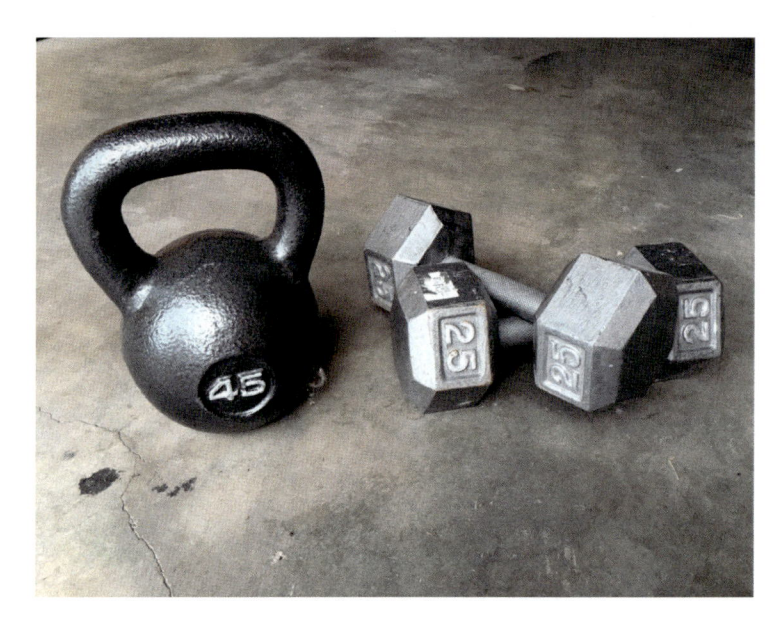

This collection of free-weights may not look like much, but they can work magic if you have the right skills.

I always recommend starting off with a simple pair of adjustable dumbbells. You can do pretty much anything with them and a simple flat bench. When you're done you can stash the bench in a corner and store the dumbbells under the bench.

For folks who like to get a little on the heavier side, a basic barbell with some weight plates will work well. Kettlebells are also a popular tool and they can be very efficient. Some people simply stash a few Kettlebells in the corner of their living room and that's their entire home gym.

Whatever weights you like to use keep in mind that it's the skills you bring to your workout that brings results, not the weights themselves. Never rely on equipment to bring results. Just as with body weight training your results depend upon how well you use your body. Not how many different ways you can work your shoulders with 3 different pieces of equipment.

5. Gymnastics rings / Suspension trainers

Another option for personal exercise is the suspension trainer. This simple device is nothing more than a couple of nylon straps with a handle on each end. They are simple, inexpensive and portable. Don't let their simplicity fool you though. Like basic free weights, a suspension trainer can replicate almost any exercise you'll ever need to do. Due to their unstable nature, you'll also add some extra challenge to common exercises you may believe are easy. Even the simple push up is new and challenging exercise when done on a set of gymnastics rings. However, even though straps or gymnastics rings can be incredibly challenging they make it very easy to adjust the level of difficulty to accommodate anyone.

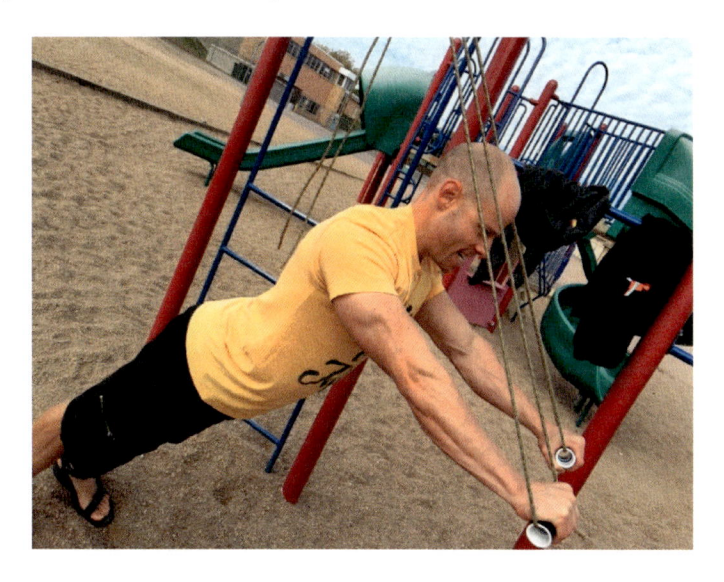

You can work your whole body with a simple pair of suspension straps.

6. Basic strength exercises

Top performers in any field know that success is achieved through mastering the basics. It seems to elude those who attempt to trick or game their fitness results with fancy yet trivial exercises. Mastering basic movements is by far the most efficient way to get the results you want. You wouldn't guess this with all of the tricks and unusual techniques out there to work every each muscle 20 different ways. Remember those strength machines sold on infomercials? The advertisements were filled with copy about how you could do 200 different exercises with a single machine.

Too many exercises eat up lifestyle resources and dilute your workout. When you spread your energy over 8 different back exercises you can only invest so much of yourself into each set and rep. This is why I highly recommend building your workout routine on a foundation of a few basic exercises. For the legs lunges and squats fit the bill. Push-ups, bench press, hand stands, overhead presses and dips work the pushing muscles. Pull ups, rows and carries work the pulling muscles. Bridges, deadlifts and kettlebell swings hit the posterior chain while sit ups and leg raises work the anterior chain. Of course, there are many variations of each of these exercises, but most variations are fairly minor influences. Use variations as needed, just make sure your squat stays a squat and the pull up is still a pull up.

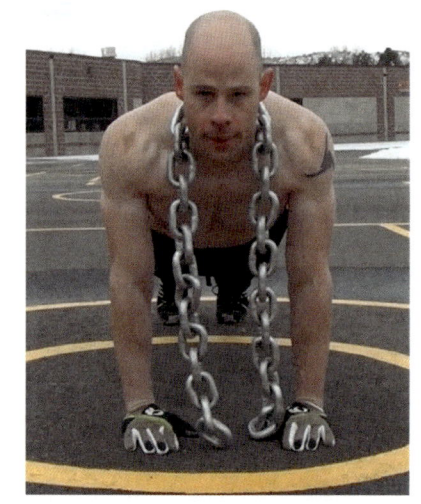

If push ups are good enough for Navy Seals they are good enough for me!

Tools of progression

It doesn't matter what you do or what tools you use. Nothing brings results without progression. Unfortunately, a lot of the most common progression methods these days are very costly such as hiring a coach or trainer or investing in special programs.

The following methods and tools will help you make progress with a fraction of the cost.

1. **Keep a workout journal**

Simply tracking what you're doing and how you're doing it will teach you volumes of personalized information. As a personal trainer, much of the value of my service comes from the simple fact that I keep a record of what people do.

You don't need to buy anything fancy. Just a simple notebook from a stationary store or even a note-taking program on your smartphone will work just fine.

2. **Smartphone fitness apps**

There are hundreds; if not thousands of inexpensive or free apps you can download right to your smart phone. These apps can help you track everything from your diet to how many steps you take, to how well you're sleeping. They can offer insight into the various influences in your life and how much impact they hold over the root cause of your goals.

While brands come and go, here are few basic apps I recommend:

- A step counting app to track how much general movement you have each day to influence your total T.E.A
- A calorie counting app to help you estimate how many calories you're consuming
- A simple workout log to track your workouts. You can also just use the simple note app that comes standard on most devices
- A camera app that allows you to watch your workout performance. An App with slow motion capabilities can teach you a lot about how you can improve your technique.

When you equip yourself with some of these simple apps, you'll be much further ahead of anyone who's simply winging their diet and exercise and hoping it all turns out well in the end.

3. **Gear- Hydration pack, shoes, clothing**

Never underestimate the importance of comfort, especially if you're going to be doing an activity outdoors. While you technically don't need any special clothing or equipment to enjoy the great outdoors, I do recommend making sure you have clothing that makes you uncomfortable. Going for a hike in jeans or wearing your motorcycle jacket on a bike ride will only hold you back.

Wearing athletic clothing that's lightweight allows more freedom of movement for your activity. If it's hot, dress lightly, wear a hat and be sure to use sunscreen. If it's cold, dress in layers and don't neglect accessories like a scarf or gloves. Remember, comfort can mean all the difference in the world towards helping you stay consistent in your habits.

I also highly recommend a backpack with a hydration system. These can make it very easy to carry water, food and anything else you'll need to stay comfortable and hydrated when exercising outside. They are also a great way to stash a suspension trainer along for a walk to the local playground.

4. **Local clubs and meet-ups**

Just because Fitness Independence means you call your own shots that doesn't mean you always have to go it alone. Making social connections can expose you to new ideas and give you fresh insight into old habits. Training with others can also be highly motivating and enjoyable plus you can learn from others who have accomplished what you want to achieve.

You don't have to join a pricey sports club either. Social apps like Meetup and even Craigslist can be great ways to discover like-minded people who enjoy doing what you want to do. Local running and cycling stores often sponsor free group rides anyone can join in on a few times a week.

5. **Books, videos and podcasts**

Your ability to progress your diet and exercise habits is heavily influenced by your knowledge and understanding. You can expect your progression to be very slow and often not happen at all if you don't open yourself to new ideas on a regular basis.

The good news is you don't have to attend college or even a single class to learn about fitness. The internet has made all of the information you'll ever need available right on your smart phone, often for free.

My first recommendation is to read. Books are difficult to produce but easy to consume. This means the information in a book has often gone through a bit more of a trial and error process so it's been tested over time. This book is a great example as I've added and removed sections based on my own learning over the past 10 years. The parts you're now reading have endured a lot of scrutiny so I've got a lot more faith in them.

The best fitness books you'll ever read are not best sellers or mentioned on talk shows. They are found in classrooms. That's right, text books, while dry and not all that exciting to read, contain some of the most honest and trustworthy information you'll ever find. The information in a text books is also not usually spun around a dogmatic ideal.

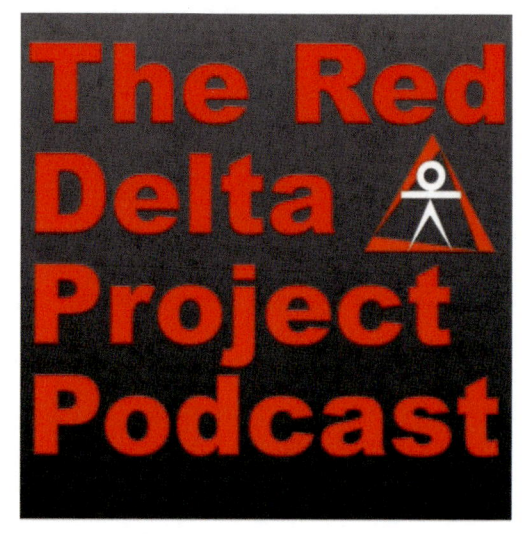

I post new information on Fitness Independence each week though the Red Delta Project Podcast

The second recommendation I have is to subscribe to fitness podcasts and YouTube videos. Information through these mediums is much cheaper and easier to produce giving you content you can consume easily. This allows a consistent flow of ideas to reach you so you can continue to grow.

DFMs for healthy eating

A lot of people are under the mistaken idea that healthy eating needs to warrant doubling their food budget. Nothing could be further from the truth! If anything, improving your diet should save you money and time.

Here are just a few resources to will help you do just that!

1. **The grocery store**

Most folks don't consider the modern day grocery store to be much of a resource for healthy eating, but it is. If you have reliable access to a fully stocked grocery store, you've got healthy resources that the kings and queens of the past couldn't have imagined. I'm not talking about those, new age "healthy" grocery stores where you can buy bottles of asparagus water for $6 and gluten free bread that's the density of a black hole. I'm referring to your run-of-the-mill grocery store that sells snack cakes, cat food, and toilet cleaning supplies all within a 30-second walk from each other.

The modern grocery store is a miracle of healthy eating and Fitness Independence. It brings a massive variety of foods under one roof and sells it all at very low prices. You can get just about anything you'll ever need to prepare whatever you enjoy 24 hours a day 7 days a week.

I feel I have to mention the grocery store here because so many people fail to make it a central part of their healthy eating plan. These days many people don't eat a lot of food from the grocery store. The wake up and grab breakfast from a coffee shop on the way to work. At work, they snack on whatever they can find in the break room or vending machines until it's time for lunch. At that point it's up to the limited options in the cafeteria or maybe lunch is grabbed at a local sandwich shop or restaurant. By the time they get out of work take-out is a tempting option or maybe they go out with friends to grab a bite to eat.

Just observe the next time you do anything outside your home that isn't work related. Go to the movies, take a road trip, attend a concert or even just go for a walk down the street. You'll witness a society that's built loads of food options so you can quickly and easily grab a bite to eat any time you like. I've even seen large churches and the local furniture store sell coffee and sandwiches.

All of these dine-out influences mean people are spending a lot of money and energy eating food they don't actually buy and prepare for themselves. In light of this, wouldn't it make sense that a store selling dietary staples like rice, chicken, fruits and vegetables seem like a more sensible alternative?

2. Your own kitchen and appliances

These days there are loads of special appliances that can make it easier to prepare your own food. I personally use one of those George Foreman Grills to cook up meat plus I have a rice cooker, a slow cooker and even a little machine that makes breakfast sandwiches. All of these things are relatively cheap and they make it easier to prepare my own food. Plus, there's the humble refrigerator and freezer. These conveniences are easy to take for granted, but they allow you the luxury of storing and preserving food. This makes cooking and preserving food a lot easier and more efficient.

What an incredible feat of modern living it is to buy or rent nearly any living quarters and it comes stocked with a dedicated space for preparing your own food! That's like the cheapest apartment rentals coming with a complete home gym! Yet, somehow people take such modern conveniences for granted and spend extra time and money to eat food they have little control over.

3. Internet cooking tips

I can understand how eating out has become so much of a trend. For one thing, it does take some time and effort to make your own food, but for those who hold the skills, a simple healthy meal can be whipped up in a few minutes. What's lacking is the skill of preparing the food. Mention home cooking to many people and they feel doomed to a diet of canned soup and simple pasta dishes.

Thankfully there's a massive trove of lessons and recipes on the Internet and it's almost all free. All you have to do is search for "15 minute healthy dinners" or "delicious ways to use ground beef" and you're golden! Everything you need to know if just a few keystrokes away.

4. Basic staples

I'm a guy who likes to stick to the basics. I really appreciate meals made with simple staple ingredients. Ground beef, chicken, salmon, fruit, mixed vegetables, rice, spices, sauces, bread, nuts and a few dairy items make up the bulk of what I eat.

What's great about all of these staples is they can be prepared and cooked in a million different ways. The basic staples are often your best value as well. You can buy meat, rice, fruit and vegetables in bulk plus it's easy to freeze these items for later. By making the basic staples the foundation of your diet, you'll prepare meals that are quicker, easier, cheaper and far tastier than what you could get at a cheap restaurant.

5. Keep a list

Nothing streamlines your life like the habit of list keeping and that's especially the case with food shopping. When you keep a grocery list you spend less, avoid impulse purchases and protect against forgetting anything at the store.

I used to roll my eyes at the idea of having a shopping list. Like keeping a workout log, it's just not sexy or fancy, but it will save you so much time and money it's crazy. Also don't worry about being confined to a list either. I like to have one or two "wild card" items on my list. That way if I want to make a couple of impulse purchases I can, but they don't overrun my shopping trip.

6. Brown bag Your Food

Making your own food goes a lot further if you can carry your lunch for the day. Even something as simple as bringing a bag of trail mix when you're going to be out for a few hours can help keep your diet and your budget in check. Plus, you won't have to look for whatever is available in the moment if you get hungry and have to settle for poor choices.

Don't forget, preparing your food ahead of time can also save you money as well. Many foods, like fruit and granola bars, don't really need any packaging and something simple like Tupperware can help you bring hot foods to heat 'n eat at the office.

7. Cook in bulk

Preparing food in bulk can save you loads of preparation time. Most of the time, it won't take much more time to make a little food as opposed to making 2-3 times as much. Making a lot of food and packing it up to quickly heat up later will make both preparing your own food and eating it much easier.

8. Order the sides or just an entree. Snack on the smallest size possible

Just because I'm a big advocate for preparing your own food that doesn't mean you shouldn't ever eat out. Heavens no! I'm all about grabbing a slice of pizza after the game or hitting a Saturday night ice cream stand.

Still, there are a few tips on how you can still keep both your diet and the check under control. The first rule I follow when eating out is I make the main course the main course. I'm not big on appetizers or filling up on bread at the table. I never quite got the reason for appetizers. It's not like the portion size of the entree won't be enough. I can't imagine a time when I've polished off a burrito at a Mexican restaurant and thought to myself "I'm still hungry, I should have started with the chips and guacamole.

When it comes to getting a treat, like some popcorn at a movie or an ice cream cone I almost always opt for the smallest size available. These days, serving sizes have grown out of control and even "medium" sizes are 2-3 times the amount you need.

I find that 99% of the time the "kids size" is plenty for me to enjoy without the risk of overeating. It's also the least expensive option as well. It's also easy for me to order the smallest size because I tell myself if that portion isn't enough then I give myself permission to go back and get more. That way I don't feel like I'm limiting myself. If I really want more I can get more.

9. Follow the stop light method

I mentioned the stop light method in the chapter on the root cause of healthy eating. To recap, green light foods are the foods that make up the bulk of your diet and you want to keep these foods ready to eat within your environment. Yellow light foods are the snacks and treats you have in small amounts and you can control your intake of these foods without too much trouble. These items you have in modest quantities in your environment and they are kept tucked away or not quite ready to eat. Red light foods are the foods you struggle to eat within healthy levels and they can quickly drain your willpower. You don't have to keep them permanently out of your diet but you do not allow them into your environment as much as possible to prevent them from becoming an issue.

A word of caution on DFMs:

The biggest issue with methods like these is they are "boring." They are not cutting edge nor are they fancy and new age. There's not a lot of excitement around them. It's not like you'll find someone proudly wearing a T-shirt telling the world they use a list when they go grocery shopping. These methods are under the radar for many people who want to get in shape, but that's why they are so great. They work within your lifestyle rather than flashier and costlier methods which bully their way into your life. You don't have to become "one of those people" to adopt these methods.

The flashy and sexy image comes from the *results* of getting in shape, not the methods you use. In these days of social media people love to adopt diet and exercise methods that look good on a Facebook post or lend themselves well to a Twitter feed. They want something they can use to make themselves feel unique and special because they belong to a club.

Fitness independence is dogma and image free. It doesn't require a secret handshake or the use of any special tools. It's simply about being in great shape on your own terms. You are your own brand. You're not part of a movement or trend but rather you're just using simple and basic methods that help you fulfill the cause of your goal as efficiently as possible. There isn't anything impressive or cool about it. *Getting* in shape isn't supposed to be cool or sexy. It's *being* in shape and owning the results you want that carry the sex appeal. After all, it's not the vehicle that matters, but the destination. Who cares if you show up to the party in an economical boring car? When you're the life of the party, everyone forgets how you got there while the shy wallflower that drove up in the red convertible fades into the crowd. So don't pass these simple methods by because they are old news and don't come with colorful packaging. I promise you they can deliver the goods for pennies on the dollar.

The end is here!

Well my friend that's it. You now have the tools, the weapons and the know how to be fit and live free. You have everything you need.

"But wait!!" I can hear you say, "What about doing cardio before strength training? Should I work out on an empty stomach to burn fat or do you think I should eat a protein shake beforehand?" "If I'm over 60 is running still good for my knees or should I look more into cycling? And my friend lost a ton of weight on a juice fast, should I try it too?" I know, there are still a lot of questions to be answered. I've probably stirred up more questions than you may have had before you started reading this book. You may even feel less certain about what to do than before. If that's the case, then I've accomplished what I set out to do.

Many fitness books attempt to give you a solid answer you can take refuge in. They promise the solution is avoiding sugar or lifting weights at a certain tempo. While these "fixes" are great for selling books, they are nothing more than another educated guess that shackles your freedom and potential.

The last thing you ever want is 100% certainty about how you should eat and exercise. Uncertainty fuels creativity and the quest for progression. It's how you learn to improve your technique or find a way to make it easier to fulfill the cause of your goal. Nothing chains you down and prevents you from growing like feeling you know for sure what you're doing. Once you know what you're doing, you stop looking for ways to progress and grow.

If you've come this far and you still have questions, that's good. It means the road is stretching out before you and discovery await your every step. You simply need to take that first step to begin. Then the next step, and the step after that. They say a journey of a thousand miles starts with a single step. It also continues with a single step and even ends with a single step. Take that step, especially if it's small and won't cost you much. That step may be nothing more than making a grocery list or planning to do ten pushups each night before bed. It doesn't have to be anything life changing. You have nothing to lose but a lot to gain and, no, you don't have to know for sure what you're doing. In fact, you probably shouldn't. The Delta Principles and root causes are not meant to be answers or solutions. They are simply a needle on a compass telling you which direction to head. How you travel is up to you. Be curious and grow. Not knowing for sure what you're doing is a beautiful thing. Don't be like so many others who wait for certainty before moving forward. If anything, certainty will probably tell you you're fine where you are and prevent you from moving forward.

As you continue to take your step, I invite you to ask questions through my email at RedDeltaProject@gmail.com. You can also browse my videos on YouTube and podcasts on iTunes, Stitcher and Google Play.

You've reached the end of this book, but the journey is just starting, or maybe it's continuing. I won't lie; there will be ups and downs. There will be times you will question everything you're doing and even yourself. These are not times of weakness, but times of opportunity to grow and learn. So I will leave off with a simple wish that even though you grow and progress, I hope this whole fitness game remains a beautiful mystery to you. There's a lot to discover and even more to enjoy.

Be Fit & Live Free,

-Matt Schifferle

Made in the USA
Monee, IL
19 December 2019